HOME TREATMENT AND POSTURE

HOME TREATMENT AND POSTURE

IN INJURY, RHEUMATISM AND OSTEOARTHRITIS

by

W. E. TUCKER

C.V.O., M.B.E., T.D., M.A., M.B., B.Ch., F.R.C.S.

Honorary Consulting Orthopaedic Surgeon, Royal London Homoeopathic Hospital; Hunterian Professor, Royal College of Surgeons, 1958, Fellow of the British Orthopaedic Association; Fellow of the Royal Society of Medicine; formerly Honorary Colonel 17th (London) General Hospital T.A.; Consulting Orthopaedic Surgeon, Royal London Homoeopathic Hospital; Orthopaedic Surgeon, Horsham and Dorking Hospitals; Registrar, Royal National Orthopaedic Hospital; Surgeon, St. John's Hospital, Lewisham; Orthopaedic Surgeon, St. John's Clinic and St. Stephen's Hospital, Fulham; Orthopaedic Surgeon, Erith Hospital.

Foreword by

PROFESSOR SIR LUDWIG GUTTMANN

C.B.E., M.D., F.R.C.P., F.R.C.S., Hon.D.Ch.

Consultant and Director of Research, National Spine Injuries Centre, Stoke Mandeville Hospital, Aylesbury; Emeritus Professor University of Cologne; President International Medical Society Paraplegia; President British and International Sports Association for the Disabled

E. & S. LIVINGSTONE LTD.

EDINBURGH AND LONDON

1969

By the same author

ACTIVE ALERTED POSTURE
1960

HOME TREATMENT IN INJURY AND OSTEOARTHRITIS
1961

PRINTED IN GREAT BRITAIN

This book is dedicated to
CHARLES STEWART MOTT
in appreciation of the great and magnificent work
and example accomplished by his Foundation in
Flint, Michigan, U.S.A.

FOREWORD

It is a great pleasure to write a Foreword to this book which I consider to be of great value for both medical practitioners and their patients. The author's philosophy in his approach to patients is firmly based on the modern principle of rehabilitation, to make the patient himself the most active member of the rehabilitation team. To achieve this it is essential to instruct the patient about details of his disability, for if he understands the nature of his complaint he certainly will be more willing to carry out verbal and written instructions given to him for his own treatment at home. In all disorders of the locomotor system the patient's concentration on his posture during his daily activities at home is of vital importance, and the author is to be congratulated for having elaborated this in such excellent detail. Mr Tucker's book rightly deserves a wide circulation amongst medical practitioners, physiotherapists, welfare officers, and above all, amongst patients.

1969.   LUDWIG GUTTMANN

PREFACE

As there was still a great demand for copies of my previous books, *Active Alerted Posture* and *Home Treatment in Injury and Osteoarthritis* when they went out of print, I decided to publish them in one volume.

The ill effects of bad posture combined with the stress and strain of every-day life inevitably take their toll. Active Alerted Posture and Home Treatment can help together to do much to avert the ageing process.

It would seem evident to me that in the individual who slumps, strain is primarily thrown on the postural muscles and, in time, on the joints which these muscles are intended to support. It would appear that one of the most important factors in the causation of muscular rheumatism and so-called fibrositis, is postural strain.

As the effects of strain progress, so the articular cartilages become worn with the onset of osteoarthritis. This is associated with disc degeneration and neuritis in the case of the spine, and osteoarthritis in weight-bearing joints.

I have become more and more impressed by the marked improvement of patients with these complaints who faithfully carry out their Home Treatment. In many cases, it is detrimental to the patients to bring them long distances for physiotherapy, because any good it may achieve is negated by the tiring effect of a tedious journey. Those patients living in outlying districts who carry out their Home Treatment regularly, often obtain better results than those living in towns, who can get physiotherapy, because the latter fail to apply themselves conscientiously to their Home Treatment. It would also seem to me, nevertheless, that Active Alerted Posture should be a *sine qua non* of all orthopaedic work. Before any operative procedure is contemplated for arthrodesing weak joints, attempts should first be made to teach the patient how to stabilise them himself by fixing and locking the joints at the various prime fixing levels before starting an action.

I should like to express my thanks to Sir Ludwig Guttmann for his generous Foreword, and once again my grateful appreciation to Mrs Audrey Besterman for her excellent drawings, and to my wife, Molly Castle, Air Commodore G. H. Dhenin, my Secretary, and Operating Sister, Miss Harper, for all their help.

Finally, I am greatly indebted to my Publishers, Messrs. E. & S. Livingstone Ltd., for advice and assistance.

1969.   W. E. TUCKER

CONTENTS

PART I

CHAPTER I

HOME TREATMENT

There are many disorders of the human body in which treatment at home by the patients themselves will go far towards hastening recovery, avoiding complications and arresting the process of physical deterioration. The improvement in certain pathological conditions of patients who have carried out home treatment conscientiously is often remarkable. Progress after operation or during a course of physiotherapy may be greatly accelerated.

In my own Orthopaedic Clinics the patients have, for some years, been given clear instructions on the home treatment appropriate to their condition. These instructions, which include descriptions of remedial exercises, were printed in separate leaflets, simply worded and illustrated, so that the patients could understand how they might expedite their own recovery. This series of leaflets attracted wide attention and I have often been asked by general practitioners if they could have them for their own patients. This gave me the idea of publishing the whole series in the form of a book so that the doctors could pass on exact instructions in each individual case.

Some of my medical readers may wonder whether it is wise to give patients clinical details of their condition. My experience has been that, in most orthopaedic conditions, it is essential to obtain the patient's co-operation. The best way to get this co-operation is to tell him the nature of his disability, its cause, the principles of the treatment and the way he can help to ensure his own recovery. This encourages him to pursue his home treatment until he is symptom free or, if the condition is a progressive one, to persevere in the knowledge that he is actively combating its tendency to deteriorate.

Although the instructions in the leaflet are comprehensive, it is important that the doctor should explain them fully to the patient, stressing the physical improvement expected. It is also essential for the doctor to review the case from time to time to satisfy himself that the patient's interest in home treatment is maintained; to ensure that the instructions are being correctly followed; and to encourage the patient to persevere, especially to attain correct balance and good posture.

In disorders of the locomotive systems, the patient will understand the nature of his complaints more readily if he has some knowledge of correct posture and elementary body mechanics; he will find the treatment more logical and will, therefore, be more likely to co-operate. At first it requires a great effort of concentration to achieve correct posture with its exacting requirements. Childhood is the best time to learn, so that proper growth may be encouraged, and the accumulative damage caused by mechanical strain may be prevented.

Good posture is an investment which brings long-term as well as immediate dividends.

CHAPTER II

INDICATIONS FOR HOME TREATMENT

Home treatment is particularly suitable for the management of muscle and joint disability arising from the following causes:

1. Postural strain: (a) everyday life
                     (b) occupational
                     (c) recreational
2. Injury
3. Degenerative condition: osteoarthritis
4. Sepsis
5. Local vascular disturbances
6. The ageing process

Postural strain

(a) **The strain of everyday life.** It is my firm belief that poor posture creates avoidable strain on certain muscles – the so-called anti-gravity muscles, especially those of the shoulder girdle, neck, spine, buttocks, thighs, knees and feet. Strain on these muscles produces tenderness and stiffness, symptoms variously ascribed to 'fibrositis', 'lumbago', 'rheumatism', or 'slipped disc'. At this stage, education in proper posture and other forms of home treatment can often effect a rapid and lasting cure.

If the muscles are not exerting their supporting influence, the underlying joints eventually begin to show the effects of joint strain and evidence of wear and tear. In the spine this condition of strain leads to spondylosis, and in weight-bearing joints such as the hip, knee and ankle, to osteoarthritis. The two conditions are similar, for spondylosis is a combination of disc degeneration and osteoarthritic change. Osteoarthritis is a wearing out of the articular cartilage. It is considered more fully later.

(b) **Occupational strain.** The effects of occupational strain often become manifest because the patient is constantly using a group of muscles and joints which are already handicapped by poor posture. The combination of both postural and occupational strains causes minor aches, stiffness and pain in many millions of people each year. Home treatment aimed at eradicating the fundamental cause – faulty posture – and other simple measures, can effect a rapid cure.

(c) **Recreational strain.** If the individual's posture is poor, if he is what I call a 'slumper', there will be a tendency for 'fibrositis', or 'rheumatism' to develop in the anti-gravity muscles. He becomes aware of a certain amount of early morning stiffness in these muscles, but the symptoms may not appear until after he has exercised. Early morning stiffness may be particularly severe after unaccustomed exercise. On the other hand, an apparently trivial injury may aggravate an existing 'rheumatism' in the muscles and produce a condition out of all proportion to the severity of the strain.

Injury

In all types of injury, particularly fractures, the disability is often prolonged by traumatic swelling, and by the loss of tone and power in the muscles of the affected region. Joint movement, also, may become limited. Suitable home treatment accelerates the absorption of the swelling, the recovery of muscle tone and the return of normal joint movement. Moreover, the gentle hyperaemia induced by frequent intervals of graduated exercises promotes callus formation and enhances the consolidation of fractures.

Osteoarthritis

The onset of osteoarthritis in a joint frequently presents itself as vague muscular aches and pains around the joint, with joint stiffness following periods of inactivity. When the joint is examined, it is usually possible to observe some limitation of movement in one or more directions, with discomfort or actual pain in the extremes of movement. These symptoms are frequently ascribed to muscular 'rheumatism', but they may be the earliest manifestation of osteoarthritis. At this stage the changes are in the articular cartilage and soft tissues around the joint and there may be nothing unusual to be seen in the radiograph. It is in such early cases that a course of home treatment, supplemented by more formal physiotherapy, can prove so rewarding. The range of movement of the joint improves, and the muscles which have become weak begin to strengthen again so that the joint becomes more stable. The stability reduces the wear and tear on the joint, prolonging its life, and reducing the patient's symptoms. In the chapter on the treatment of osteoarthritis, I have specified five categories of local treatment according to the response to therapy. In the first three categories, conservative treatment consists of a basic regime of home treatment together with specific measures, the choice of which depends on the severity of the symptoms.

Septic conditions

After the healing of any septic process, whether of the soft tissues, bone or joint, there may be residual stiffness of the part, and rigidity of the soft tissues may limit the movement of a joint, even though the joint itself has not been infected. Home treatment helps to restore the part involved to normal function.

Vascular disturbances

The blood supply to a part of the body may be reduced suddenly, as when an artery is blocked by an embolus; or gradually, as in the progressive narrowing of vessels in endarteritis or arteriosclerosis. Whatever the degree of vascular disturbance, home treatment, by encouraging the collateral circulation, helps to minimise the damage.

The ageing process

In the normal ageing process, many of the tissues, particularly the superficial ones, become tender even to the slightest touch. This tenderness is thought to be due to a collection of waste products or metabolites in relatively avascular areas. Home treatment, by improving the blood flow, helps to disperse these waste products, and hence to alleviate the symptoms.

This, then, is a brief description of the conditions in which home treatment can play an important part in the patient's recovery. Home treatment provides the continuous therapy that he needs; for out-patient physiotherapy, excellent though it is, suffers from the drawback that it is inevitably sporadic.

CHAPTER III

POSTURE

It is my belief that the posture of the individual is of the utmost importance. I want now to make clear what I mean by good posture, and why it is so vital.

Most people accept their acquired posture without conscious thought. The posture developed in early childhood usually remains unchanged throughout life, whether it is good or bad. Yet a really correct posture is rewarding not only to health but to appearance. It can also delay the degenerative process of the ageing body.

I have found in many years of orthopaedic practice that people who continuously – if unconsciously – adopt a slumped posture tend to develop a number of avoidable body ills, and are less positive in their approach to life. It has become clear to me that a more dynamic attitude towards posture yields positive results. My studies and observations have led me to adopt the concept of **'Active, Alerted Posture'**, a simple postural guide which can nevertheless profoundly influence health and bodily efficiency.

Once the principles of **Active, Alerted Posture** have been understood, and put into practice, the body is at all times prepared for any sort of action. Correct posture helps to reduce accidents in the home, industry, travel and sport by ensuring a greater precision in action and it helps to avoid, or at least to delay, the effects of the osteoarthritic process, which may follow upon an injury.

Correct upright posture is the consequence of a particular attitude of the mind towards the body; one which promotes both mental and physical equilibrium and poise. Once the principles have been accepted and mastered, the various positions can be held unconsciously with little exertion. There will be no sign of tension and no wasted effort. It is balanced posture, and therefore, is a form of continuous isometric exercise, since the muscles on one side of the body are constantly working against those of the opposite side.

The development of the upright posture. In infancy, children are recumbent, offering no resistance to gravity but as their pyramidal tracts develop they are able to stand upright. Learning to walk is a gradual process, usually preceded by crawling. By degrees, balance improves and a child learns to toddle, beginning with a few timorous, experimental steps. As balance is mastered, standing and walking become a habit.

Some children adopt the correct upright posture naturally, others need to be taught and, ultimately, are able to maintain the correct attitude continuously, without thinking about it. Childhood is the best time to learn but it is a simple matter for older people also to master the correct upright posture and derive physical benefit as a result.

Skeletal types. Obviously everybody is not built in the same mould; each of us has different structure and different bone formation. Yet the general shape of the skeleton is such that,

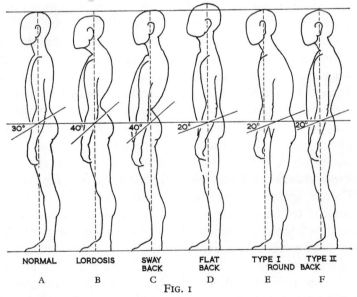

NORMAL	LORDOSIS	SWAY BACK	FLAT BACK	TYPE I ROUND BACK	TYPE II
A	B	C	D	E	F

FIG. 1

The average skeletal type and four defective skeletal types (After Wiles).

when they stand, most people assume a similar posture. In this average skeletal type, the pelvic inclination is 30° (Fig. IA) and the line of gravity of the body passes vertically through the mastoid process, down through the shoulder joint, and in front of the sacro-iliac joint, the knee joint and the ankle joint. But there are variations. Wiles (1959), for instance, described these as due to two components:

1. an increase or decrease in the pelvic inclination, or
2. dorso-lumbar kyphosis.

These two variables combine to produce four defective skeletal types:

(a) the lordotic back: distinguished by an increase in the pelvic inclination, the dorso-lumbar spine being mobile (Fig. IB),

(b) the sway back: also with an increase in the pelvic inclination, combined with a dorso-lumbar kyphosis (Fig. IC),

(c) the flat back: there is a decrease in the pelvic inclination, but the dorso-lumbar spine is mobile (Fig. ID),

(d) the round-shouldered back: the pelvic inclination is diminished, but there is a dorso-lumbar kyphosis (Figs. IE and F).

The line of gravity varies according to the skeletal type.

Postural attitudes. Three postural attitudes, however, can be adopted by any skeletal type, whether it is the normal back, the lordotic back, the flat back, the sway back, or the round-shouldered back.

These three attitudes apply not only to the upright body, but also when it is sitting or lying. They are:

1. **Active, Alerted.** This is the most efficient attitude, when the body is upright, but also as a preliminary to movement from any position (Fig. 2). This is posture in balance (Chap. IV).

2. **Inactive, Slumping.** This is the commonest attitude of all. A slumping, inactive posture is inefficient, whether a person is standing, sitting or lying (Fig. 3). This is unbalanced posture.

3. **Passive Support.** At rest, when sitting or lying, the body is supported (by chair, bed, couch or pillows) with the joints in a

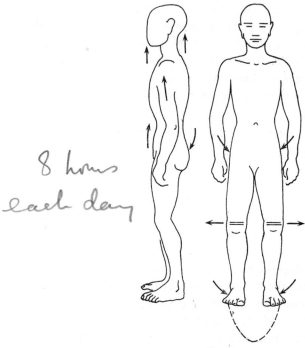

*8 hours
each day*

FIG. 2

Active Alerted Posture is also balanced, concentric posture. Muscles on opposite
sides of the body are in slight isometric contraction.

neutral position (Figs. 4 and 5). This is the proper posture of
relaxation.

In the upright position only the first two attitudes are possible.
In the sitting or lying positions, all three are possible.

Skeletal structures. The skeletal structures consist of bones
joined together by ligaments, acted on and controlled by muscles,
and influenced by gravity unless suitably supported in the sitting
or recumbent positions. The mechanism of **Active Alerted
Posture** is easy to understand if the body is considered as a series
of mobile sections articulating at six main prime fixing levels
(Fig. 6).

1. The first level is at the ankle-joint and foot. The ankles and
feet form two firm bases, on which falls the entire weight of the

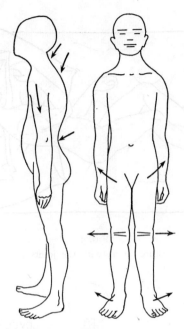

FIG. 3

Inactive Slumping Posture is also unbalanced, eccentric posture. Gravity strains are not prevented.

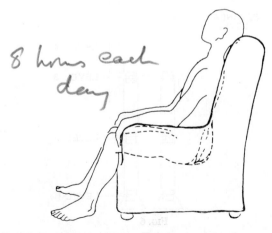

8 hours each day

FIG. 4

Passive Supported Posture; sitting with the joints in neutral position.

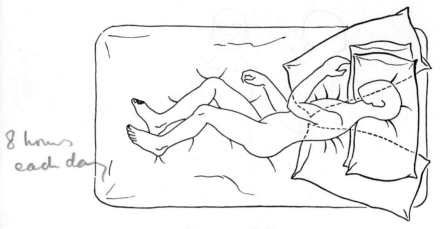

8 hours each day

FIG. 5

Passive Supported Posture; lying with the joints in a neutral position.

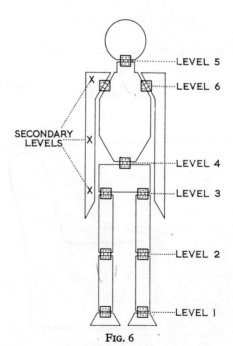

FIG. 6

The six main prime fixing levels of the body with secondary levels at wrist, elbow and shoulder joints.

body. When a man stands, the ankle and feet should be locked by the balanced action of the muscles, so that the whole weight of the body is transmitted through the talus to the hard bony outer side of the foot, formed by the os calcis, cuboid and fifth metatarsal bones.

2. The second level is at the knee. This joint acts as a shock absorber. If the muscles are in balanced contraction, the knees being slightly bent, the weight of the body above is prevented from falling directly on the joint ligaments and bony components.

3. The third level is at the hip joint. The pelvis, with the trunk, upper limbs, and head is supported on the heads of each femur at the hip joints. The weight of the body is transmitted from the pelvis to the femoral shafts via the head and neck of each femur.

4. The fourth level is at the lumbo-sacral articulations. The whole weight of the upper extremities, head and trunk, is transmitted from the vertebral column at the lumbo-sacral articulations to the sacrum and thence through the sacro-iliac joints to the pelvis. The pelvis is greatly thickened, in the area between the sacro-iliac joint and the acetabulum, owing to the transference of the body weight.

5. The fifth level is where the head joins the neck. Pure flexion and extension of the head on the neck, as in nodding, takes place at the occipito-atlantoid articulations. In normal flexion and extension of the head and neck, most of the movement occurs between the fifth and sixth vertebrae.

6. The sixth level is at the attachments of the upper limbs to the trunk at the shoulder girdle. The girdle, consisting of the clavicle and the scapula, attaches the limb to the trunk anteriorly by a synovial joint, the sternoclavicular joint. In addition, the girdle is fixed to the body by a series of muscles which attach it to the base of the skull above, the iliac crest below, the vertebral column and the thoracic wall.

Other secondary levels such as the wrist, elbow, and shoulder joints, might be included but, for simplification, let us confine ourselves to the six main levels. Each of these sections is firmly attached to the next at its corresponding articulations by capsular structures and associated muscles: each section supports the one above it, like the floors of a multi-storey building, from the foundations to the topmost storey. Note that the prime fixing levels are relative to the body's position. These six are relative to the upright position: if the position is changed the prime fixing levels are also changed. In a 'hand-stand', for example, they would be those of the upper extremities, the hand and wrist, with the elbows, shoulder and shoulder girdle.

The mechanics of joint equilibrium. An object can remain stable only if the line of gravity falls within the area of its base or contact with the ground. In man, the line of gravity must fall within the area outlined by his feet when he stands without support (Fig. 7).

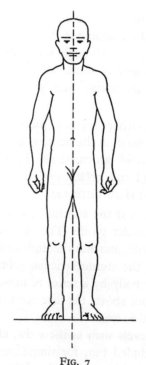

FIG. 7

Symmetrical standing in Active Alerted Posture. The body weight passes between the bony outer side of both feet.

A joint can be stable only if there is equilibrium between the forces acting on it (Steindler, 1955). Thus a balance must exist between the groups of muscles around the joint. If only a single muscle group acts, it must produce a turning effect at the joint and, unless it is counterbalanced by an equal and opposite force, will induce movement. Accordingly, the maintenance of upright posture depends on a balance between the opposing groups of muscles round each joint. The muscles are then contracting without shortening (isometric contraction).

But equilibrium is possible even when one muscle group alone contracts, if the opposing force is gravity: the balance is between gravity and muscle activity. In the upper extremity, for example, the weight of the arm and shoulder girdle act downwards on the shoulder girdle muscles: unless these contract slightly to support the arm and shoulder girdle, there will be a passive strain on the shoulder girdle muscles.

Moreover, equilibrium at a joint is possible without any muscle action whatever, if the force of gravity on one side is balanced by tension in ligaments on the other. For example, it is possible to stand with the line of the centre of gravity in front of the knee joint, and with the muscle groups round the joint relaxed, so long as there is a balance between the force of gravity acting in front of the joint and the tension in both the capsule and deep fascia behind. The hamstrings and quadriceps muscles can both be completely relaxed, provided the centre of gravity is not too far in front of the joint (Fig. 8). If, however, the arms are raised forward, the movement shifts the centre of gravity still more in front of the knee joint, and the hamstring muscles then contract to aid the capsule in maintaining equilibrium at the joint (Joseph & Nightingale, 1954). Such a posture is maintained at the cost of tension in a ligament. It quickly causes pain, and the strain on the joint structures leads eventually to real joint degeneration. It is an example of inactive slumping posture.

When two forces are exerted on opposite sides of the joint, the mechanical system is called a lever of the first order (Fig. 9A). On the other hand, when the two opposing forces are on the same

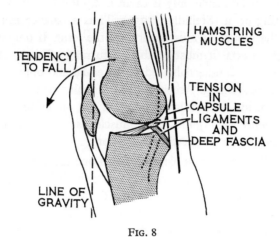

FIG. 8

Equilibrium at the knee joint.

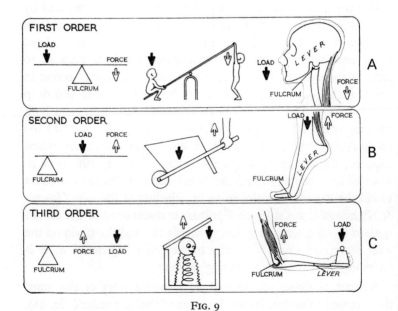

FIG. 9

The different orders of lever action in the body.

side of the joint, and therefore are attached to the same lever arm, they can only maintain equilibrium by acting in opposite directions. This is an example of the second or third order of levers (Fig. 9B and C), depending on which force is considered the primary force and which the resisting force: when the load or resisting force is nearer the joint, the lever is of the second order: when the load is farther from the joint than the primary force, this is a lever of the third order. This lever of the third order is the system which is commonly used for directing movement of the body.

The maintenance of posture depends to a greater or lesser extent on two factors: first the balanced activity of the muscles as in **Active Alerted Posture**; second the tension in the capsule and fascia round each joint, as in Inactive Slumping Posture.

The classical idea, based on the work of Sherrington (1900), that the postural muscles are all in a continuous state of reflex activity needs to be modified. Postural muscles can relax completely when passive forces in the ligaments are available and strong enough to take over the task of supporting or counterbalancing the force of gravity: but it is an unnatural state which in time promotes degenerative change in the joint structures.

Another established idea – that the ligaments and surrounding fascia of a joint are completely inextensible, i.e. that they only become taut at the extreme limit of movement of joint – should be modified in view of recent investigations into the passive mechanisms which stabilise joints. The fully extended position of a joint is not an absolute and limiting position. Passive tensions arise in and around the joint before the ultimate limit of movement occurs (particularly at the knee) and can play a major role in supporting the body against the force of gravity, even though the joint is not at the limit of movement (Fig. 8). It is often argued that ligaments can play no part in maintaining posture because taut ligaments become rapidly painful. When one rests the heels on a railway carriage seat, for example, one feels pain behind the knees. But the pain is not immediate: it seldom appears for at least half a minute. When a man stands, he makes constant small changes of position, at average intervals of about half a minute, and consequently the ligaments are never stretched for a long enough period to become consciously painful before the tension is relieved. It may be that when the ligaments do in fact begin to signal their resentment, the first signals are appreciated at a subconscious level, so that position is changed by reflex action. Thus the tension is relieved before one becomes conscious of any painful sensation.

In patients with congenital absence of pain this protective mechanism is inoperative and it is a fact that their weight-bearing joints may become progressively disorganised, as in a Charcot's joint. Such patients, apart from insensitiveness to pain, have a normal nervous system.

The centre of gravity of the body. The centre of gravity is through the sacral prominence at the level of the second sacral

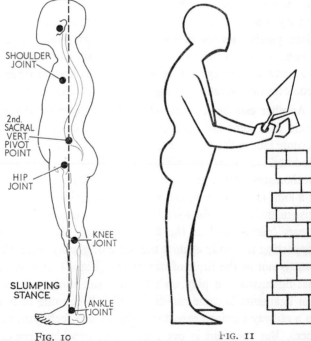

FIG. 10

Non-alignment of line of gravity forces in Inactive Slumping Posture.

FIG. 11

Non-alignment of line of gravity forces in Inactive Slumping Posture is like a badly built brick wall.

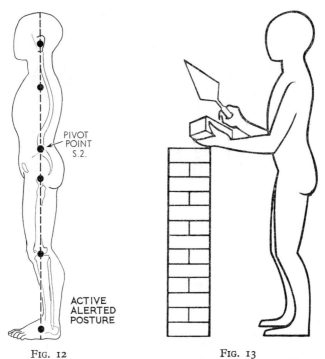

PIVOT
POINT
S.2.

ACTIVE
ALERTED
POSTURE

FIG. 12   FIG. 13
Correct alignment of line of gravity   Alignment of line of gravity forces in
forces in Active Alerted Posture.   Active Alerted Posture is like a well
                                        constructed brick wall.

vertebra. The centre of gravity of the mobile parts above, that
is to say the head on the neck, and the arms and shoulder on the
trunk, should be in a direct line. In the same way the pivot point
of the hip joint, knee and feet should be on a straight line passing
directly through the centre of the hip, knee and mid-tarsal joints.
It can be seen in Figures 10 and 11 that in the position of Inactive
Slumping Posture the various points of pivot, in the six prime
fixing levels described, are off centre; whereas in the position of
Active Alerted Posture (Figs. 12 and 13), each one is directly
above or below the centre of the body. In movement, we see that
the force, the load and the lever must be as nearly as possible
one above the other. The right and wrong ways to lift are illustrated
in Figure 14. We also see that, in any action, this can be achieved

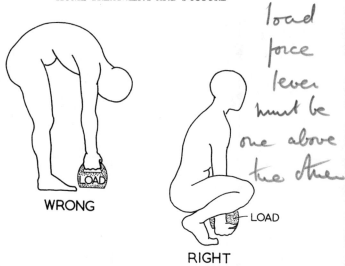

load
force
lever
must be
one above
the other

WRONG

RIGHT

FIG. 14
The right way and the wrong way to lift weights.

only if the activators work with the aid of the synergists on the firm prime fixing muscles at the prime fixing level. This is illustrated in Figures 15 and 16.

It appears, then, that the upright posture can be, and probably in many people is, maintained with remarkably little muscle activity except for the continuous activity of the erector spinae to maintain the posture of the spine. All other muscle groups may be largely without muscle tone and only come into activity to control larger postural swaying movements. In this inactive slumping posture, the joints of the body are not in a perfect, balanced position because the general line of gravity is either in front or behind each joint. This means that the weight of the body must be counterbalanced to a large extent by passive tension in the joint tissues. The price to be paid is threefold. First, when the stress on the supporting ligaments exceeds a certain time limit, damage results, and this becomes progressive over the years. Second, perhaps more important still, abnormal shocks or strains are transmitted directly to the joint, since the inactive or poorly contracting muscles afford little protection. (Consider the back as

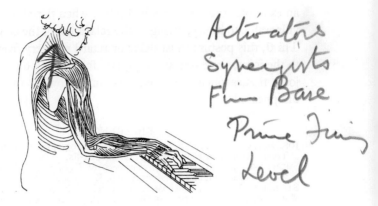

Activators
Synergists
F___ Base
Prime Fix__
Level

FIG. 15

Pianist in the act of playing showing the activating groups of muscles controlling the fingers, the synergistic groups controlling the wrist, elbow and shoulder joints, and the prime fixor groups controlling the shoulder girdle.

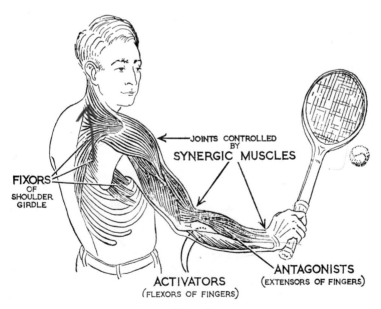

JOINTS CONTROLLED BY
SYNERGIC MUSCLES

FIXORS OF SHOULDER GIRDLE

ANTAGONISTS
(EXTENSORS OF FINGERS)

ACTIVATORS
(FLEXORS OF FINGERS)

FIG. 16

To demonstrate how the correctly executed backhand tennis shot is performed by activators acting in conjunction with synergists and prime fixors.

an example: the lumbar spinal joints when flexed are exceedingly vulnerable to injury, owing to the relaxation of the erector spinae.) Third, this posture must delay or retard recovery from any injury to the joint, since stresses of gravity fall directly on the recovering joint tissues once the muscle spasm following the damage has disappeared.

REFERENCES

JOESPH, J. & NIGHTINGALE, A. (1954). Electromyography of Muscles of Posture: Thigh Muscles in Males. *J. Physiol.* **126**, 81-85.
SHERRINGTON, C. S. (1900). In *Textbook of Physiology*. Ed. Schafer, E A., vol. II Edinburgh and London: Young J. Pentland.
STEINDLER, A. (1955). *Kinesiology*. Springfield, Illinois: Thomas.
WILES, P. (1959). *Essentials of Orthopaedics*. 3rd ed. London: Churchill.

CHAPTER IV

THE PRACTICAL APPLICATION OF ACTIVE ALERTED POSTURE

Rudolph Magnus said (1926) 'Posture is an active process, and is the result of a great number of reflexes, many of which have a tonic character'.

I come now to a description of **Active Alerted Posture.**

The entire body on the feet and ankles

Firm, resilient support of the human frame stems from the ability to stand firmly on both feet, with the joints of the feet and ankles stabilised by muscle action, like a house built on a solid foundation of rock.

The human foot has two functions to perform – the static or supporting function at rest and the dynamic function during movement.

In the static phase the weight of the body should be taken evenly on the heel and the outer side of the foot; the toes should also be brought into the action of standing so that pressure is taken off the heads of the metatarsals. Each foot has been likened to a half dome, the two feet together forming a complete one (Jones, 1949). The inner longitudinal arch of each foot is maintained by the contraction of the anterior and posterior tibial muscles and the long flexors of the toes. At the same time the toes grip the ground by the action of the short flexors and intrinsic muscles. The knee joint, held very slightly flexed, is stabilised by the balanced contraction of all the muscles, the quadriceps, the hamstrings, the abductors and adductors of the thigh. This position of feet and knees is taught to the parachutist in order that he may land smoothly and avoid injury.

If the feet are held in the flat valgus position, the one naturally adopted by the majority, there is an abduction opening

25

strain on the inner side of the knee; in Active Alerted Posture a slight adduction compressing force is produced, closing the articular surface of the femur and tibia together on the inner side of the knee. This effect is beneficial, allowing the line of gravity to pass through the centre of the knee joint.

The architect, designing a house, causes two forces of stress to meet at a point, as in a Gothic arch: one side supports the other. Thus, in Active Alerted Posture, the body weight should be taken on the outer side of the foot, pressing against the ground to form an inverted Gothic arch (Fig. 17). It was

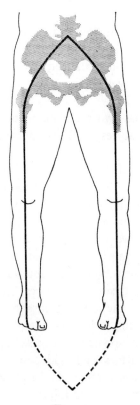

FIG. 17
Weight on the outer side of foot, with pressure against the ground; the inverted Gothic arch.

Mesendieck who stressed the importance of taking the weight on the outer side of both feet, so that the line of the forces of strain follows the gentle curves of a parabola, meeting at a point some twelve inches below the ground.

The pelvis on the hip joints

The fixation of the pelvis on the hip must be maintained by a balanced contraction of the flexors and extensors of the hip on the one hand, and the abductors and adductors on the other. Harrison *et al.* (1953) and Denham (1959) have shown that the femoral head can be likened to a nut inside a nut-cracker. It is subjected to compression, in hyperextension of the thigh, by the long lever of the femoral shaft and the anterior ligament plus the front of the acetabulum: but when there is a balanced contraction of the muscles and the joint is held actively in slight flexion, this 'nut-cracker' effect is diminished. The essential factor is to keep the glutei contracted with the other muscles surrounding the joint falling into balanced contraction. The glutei should contract so hard that a coin can be held between the natal cleft.

The trunk on the pelvis

In the slumped posture it is possible to maintain the trunk in the upright position with remarkably little muscular activity: in **Active Alerted Posture** there must be a balanced contraction of all abdominal muscles with a balanced contraction of the erectores spinae.

In **Active Alerted Posture,** flexion of the spine at the lumbo-sacral joint is performed by active contraction of the abdominal muscles, the erectores spinae working as active antagonists (co-contraction) throughout the entire movement.

The contracted abdominal muscles act as a buffer or brake to flexion. Thus, a wall of contracting muscle cushions any ill-effects that follow flexion of the spine, particularly on the fronts of the intervertebral discs.

It is important to remember that a slight active flexion position should be adopted, to decrease the lumbar curve and straighten the back, with the buttock muscles contracted and tucked under. A neutral position is then established in which no strain is imposed on any one particular vertebral structure.

The head on the neck

The head could fall into any position unless maintained upright by balanced muscle contraction. Magnus and Sherrington have postulated that the head and neck position exerts a controlling reflex action on the entire body. The chin must be kept well tucked in and the back of the neck stretched, so that the person stands to his full height.

The shoulder girdles

There must be a fixation of the shoulder girdles by continuous muscle activity, so as to oppose the downward sagging force of gravity. In slumped posture, the various muscles supporting the girdle are relaxed, and the limb sags, putting strain on the components of the cervical brachial plexus and the subclavian vessels.

In **Active Alerted Posture** the upper limbs must be held slightly elevated and, if anything, slightly forward, ensuring balanced contraction between the trapezii, levators anguli scapulae, the scalenes, rhomboids and the serrati. This prevents compression of the nerve components and the great vessels between the clavicle and first rib.

Active Alerted Posture is not simply a form of exercise to be practised occasionally: if it is to confer its full benefit, it must be held continuously, until it becomes, in fact, a tonic reflex action. At first it will require a great deal of effort and attention: just as the pianist, the ballerina, the acrobat, the athlete, work unceasingly to achieve a perfection which looks effortless, so it is necessary to persevere with **Active Alerted Posture** until the execution becomes automatic. The task may not appear so onerous to those who saw, on the television screen, the remarkable example of the woman born without arms. By persistent practice, she had taught herself to sew with the feet and to do all the sewing for her family of six children. So developed were the intrinsic muscles of her feet, that she could thread a needle with her toes.

Apart from the challenge of the necessary persistence, some patients have specific difficulties in training to maintain the posture during movement. They find it hard to walk on the outer side of the feet and to grip with the toes; and it may be useful to them to think of the foot in this position as a bow, drawn tight to shoot an arrow, and so taut with potential energy (Fig. 18).

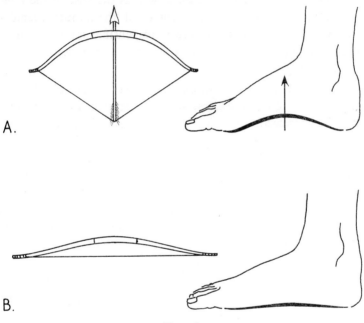

FIG. 18

A. The well supported arch of the foot with the weight carried on the bony outer side of the foot and the toes gripping the floor is likened to the tense bow.
B. The flat foot is likened to the slack bow.

Others find it hard to keep the abdominal muscles drawn in as they talk, or make a movement. They may be re-assured: what the singer and the mannequin have achieved, so can they. When they walk holding this posture, they move in a state of perfectly synchro-nised body movement. The head, neck, trunk and pelvis are held together firmly, as the upper arm of a lever. The fulcrum passes through the hip joints; and as each leg thrusts forward, pivoting from the hip, side sway and roll are almost eliminated: movement is forward, without unnecessary diversion into irrelevant directions.

To hold the abdominal muscles up against the posterior abdominal wall and still to breathe and talk is difficult at first. One must learn to use the necessary thoracic and shoulder-girdle breathing muscles in order to expand the lung bases, which so often are never properly aerated. This part of the body, containing the lower dorsal spinal muscles, as well as the base of the lungs, is a relatively immobile part – what I call 'the no man's land' of the body. Poor movement here is responsible for many of the chest complications which follow abdominal operation.

Man, of course, is not a mere physical specimen; and many of his troubles stem from the mind. There is an inter-play between mental and physical factors, so that disturbances of the mind may be expressed in physical symptoms; and disturbances of the body have their effect on the mind. It is not surprising, therefore, that improvement in the posture can have a beneficial effect on those suffering from depression. Whether it is initially the depression which produces a slumping posture, or the strains of a slumping posture which lead to depression, it may not be possible to say in an individual case: but training in Active Alerted Posture can break what may be a vicious circle and lead to both physical and mental amelioration.

I urged, in an earlier chapter, that **Active Alerted Posture** should be taught as soon as possible in childhood, as a great preventive measure against wear and tear. Other opportunities will present themselves, for example when a patient complains of any 'rheumaticky' pain, or of any injury. One most important occasion is as preliminary training for operation on a bone or joint. In my opinion this is almost mandatory, since postural training will have a profound influence on the eventual success of the operation. Once the patient has been shown the fundamentals, whether by personal instruction or by the appropriate leaflet, he can carry on at home, until Active Alerted Posture becomes a way of life.

So much for the question of *when* it is to be taught: but *who* is to introduce children and patients to so desirable a way of life?

Since Active Alerted Posture is primarily a prophylaxis and secondarily a therapy, I suggest that it is first the affair of general practitioners, schools' medical officers and physical training instructors. These are the guardians of the children's health, and the ones who can raise the physical standards of the nation. Secondly, it is the affair of doctors, orthopaedic surgeons, physiotherapists and trainers – those, in short, who are concerned with patients, young and old, and special groups like athletes.

Active Alerted Posture is by no means a panacea; but it is a method of hygiene, in the proper sense of the word, easily taught, easily learned, and, when learned and practised, of remarkable physical and mental benefit throughout life.

REFERENCES

DENHAM, R. A. (1959). Hip mechanics. *J. Bone Jt Surg.* **41B**, 550-57.
HARRISON, M. H. M., SCHAJOWICS, F. & TRUETA, J. (1953). Osteoarthritis of the hip: a study of the nature and evolution of the disease. *J. Bone Jt Surg.* **35B**, 598-626.
JONES, F. W. (1949). *Structure and Function as seen in the Foot.* 2nd ed. London: Bailliere, Tindall & Cox.
MAGNUS, R. (1926). Physiology of posture. *Lancet*, **2**, 531, 585.

CHAPTER V

THE EFFECTS OF BAD POSTURE

A patient accustomed to Inactive Slumping Posture who makes a sudden movement, may often produce an acute strain of muscles or sprain of a joint. As previously suggested, a latent morbidity may also exist in the muscles and joints as the result of Inactive Slumping Posture: any aggravation of this by reason of an injury may produce physical signs and symptoms out of all proportion to the severity of the injury. Although this may be a surmise, a careful consideration of the history of the injury, the physical signs and symptoms and the patient's postural attitude may make the impression a certainty.

Bad posture is an impossible handicap for an athlete. As the standards rise, as the competition becomes stronger, as training methods become more scientific and rigorous, the poor co-ordination of muscle movement associated with poor posture is a factor retarding performance and predisposing to injury. Athletes to-day have to possess a working knowledge of the physiology and mechanics of muscle action and the application of these to posture and movement, and they study every movement and analyse it by the techniques of kinesiology. This separates each action into its component parts, and relates it to the various types of lever action. For example, in the act of moving from one leg to another, the muscles of the foot on the ground are braced and contracted from the moment of impact, remaining so until the activators of that leg have driven the body forward. Subsequently, the moment the leg leaves the ground, there should be abeyance of all muscular activity in it, until the muscles of the other leg have activated and the first leg again becomes the fixing one. In such actions as bowling in cricket or pitching in baseball the athlete 'winds himself up', during which time the point of balance is constantly altering its position. Finally, just before the ball is released, forward movement is checked for a moment, the action being completed on a firm, rigid base, with the result that the recoil and resulting force is maximum. In this action there is thus a constant and continuous flow of movement until the movement is suddenly and abruptly checked. In jumping in the line-out in rugby, or in heading a football, the player runs the risk of knee injury unless he lands on his feet in the correct way on the outer side of the forefoot, gradually sinking on to the heels; so that eventually the landing foot becomes firmly fixed on the ground and the body weight evenly distributed over the whole of the outer weight-bearing part of the foot. By this means there is a stable base on which, by the balancing actions of the controlling muscles, the knees can bend slightly but remain under firm co-ordinated muscle control. This prevents any abnormal strain being thrown on the ligaments of the joint, particularly on its inner side.

The danger of poor posture is that the player's muscles are not ready for the movement, which begins off balance, as it were, and never achieves co-ordination. An example of the effects of unco-ordinated movement is that of two international fast bowlers who sustained identical injuries on the same day: a tear of the left abdominal obliques at their costal attachments. The first bowler, seen in the morning, stated that when he was about to deliver the ball his left foot, the forward fixing foot, slipped. The other bowler, seen in the afternoon, explained that he had mis-timed his action and delivered the ball before his left foot was firmly fixed on the ground. In both cases an activating movement had taken place on an unstable base, thus throwing a strain on the left abdominal obliques.

A wrist joint affected by a recent injury or arthritis will often give rise to pain on sudden movement because the wrist joint itself takes part in the activating movement. If, however, the joint is firmly locked by the contraction of the wrist joint fixing muscles, and the prime fixing level is transferred from the shoulder girdle level to that of the wrist joint itself, laxity and play between the joint surfaces are prevented. The same effective movement

C

can now be carried out without pain by means of the fingers working on a stable base, the wrist joint.

I have defined postural strain as the dead weight of the mobile parts on the muscles and joints associated with the fixed parts. This is the result of lack of proper muscle activity. In Inactive Slumping Posture, the pumping action of the muscles which constitutes the peripheral venous heart, is also less efficient. The return to the heart of venous blood, lymph and tissue fluid is less complete, resulting in accumulation of fluid in the extremities, particularly the lower limbs. This occurs in people who sit for a prolonged period with their feet down, as for instance on an overnight journey in a train or aeroplane, when oedema of the ankles and feet may develop. If the sciatic nerve is involved in an injury, there may be oedema of the limb, partly due to the loss of vasomotor activity in the blood vessels, but also to the slowing down of the pumping action of the muscles on the venous and lymphatic circulations. A further example of the effects of loss of muscle activity is the patient who has been confined to bed during a prolonged illness. He may show marked swelling of the legs when he gets up, and this does not resolve until vasomotor activity in the muscles has returned.

In occupational and postural strains the antigravity muscles become fatigued and strained and show areas of spasm. This makes them painful and tender. They lose their resilience, become inefficient, and no longer adequately support their underlying joints. These, in turn, suffer from strain and eventually develop degenerative changes.

A number of histological studies have been made on these tender muscles, and their supporting and overlying tissues, but in most cases these have shown no abnormality: but the techniques of electromyography have disclosed the presence of small scattered areas of spasm. It is well known that muscle in spasm is painful and tender.

Two explanations of this muscle spasm are possible: one that the spasm is produced by nerve root irritation from the adjacent strained spinal joints: the other that the muscle is fatigued, with a consequent local accumulation of metabolites. Whichever is the correct explanation, it is likely that poor posture is the initial factor which brings about this muscular tenderness. This syndrome, which has been variously called fibrositis, muscular rheumatism or myalgia, may be studied by histochemical techniques, which are correlated with the study of function; so that a comprehensive investigation has three dimensions: function, chemical composition and structure. It is possible to detect chemical changes, in muscles whose function is abnormal, before any histological change is evident. This reinforces my clinical impression, gained from experience of thousands of cases, that in the early stages of postural strain something accumulates in the tissues, resulting in pain and tenderness. As there are no structural changes at this stage, the condition can be checked, the tenderness of the muscles made to disappear, and a complete cure achieved.

Changes in the capsular ligaments of the joints

It is usually accepted that the degenerative changes associated with the wear and tear of osteoarthritis occur first of all in the articular cartilage: but this assumption may be due to the fact that the patient's symptoms are sufficiently severe to warrant operative investigation only when cartilage has become eroded. But changes are also present in the synovial membrane and the joint capsule: and it may well be that, as the result of postural strain, the first changes to develop are those in the capsule and synovia of joints, causing pain and tenderness in these structures and even effusion into the joint cavity.

Changes in cartilage and bone

Changes in the articular cartilage, and later in the subchondral bone, probably occur after the soft tissue changes. Thus the order of the involvement is muscle, capsule, synovia, cartilage. In my view postural strain evokes biochemical changes in the muscles, and, if these are not treated, further changes follow in the capsule, synovia and articular cartilage.

Once changes in the joint structures have occurred, the muscles may be further involved by a reflex protective spasm. This spasm functions as a protective mechanism to guard the joint from further strain. The spasm may involve a single group of muscles on one side of the joint, as in a sciatic scoliosis: but if the joint changes are more general, all the muscles around the joint may go into spasm. Muscle pain and tenderness may therefore occur at three distinct phases: first, in the early stages of postural strain as abnormal metabolites accumulate: second, at a later stage when the joint tissues themselves become involved, as a painful protective spasm which may occur either suddenly or gradually: and finally, when the articular changes of osteoarthritis are established, as tender, painful, fibrotic, degenerative changes in the muscles surrounding the joint involved. Thus bad posture and postural strain initiate a series of biochemical and structural changes which end in osteoarthritis. There are, of course, many other predisposing or contributory factors: injury, sepsis, toxins – bacterial or metabolic – thrombosis of the vessels around the joint, alteration of the oestrogen/androgen balance, and even constitutional hereditary factors, all of which may play an important part in the production of joint degeneration. But chronic postural strain, resulting from bad posture, is a preventable factor and one that can affect people of any age. Since Goldthwait pointed this out as far back as 1915, it merits urgent action on the widest possible scale.

The detrimental effects of bad posture on muscles and joints at the various prime fixing levels are tabulated below (Fig. 19):

Ankles and feet

Muscular : Strain of the long and short muscles of the longitudinal and transverse arches of the foot. Tenovaginitis of the tibialis posticus and anticus, flexor hallucis longus and the peroneii.

Joints : Hallux valgus. Hallux rigidus. Osteoarthritis of the mid-tarsal joints.

Bones : Stress fractures of the metatarsal bones.

Nerve involvement : Morton's metatarsalgia due to false neuroma formation in digital nerves.

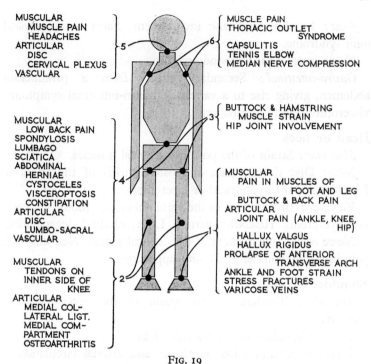

MUSCULAR
    MUSCLE PAIN
    HEADACHES
ARTICULAR
    DISC
    CERVICAL PLEXUS
VASCULAR
⎬ 5

MUSCLE PAIN
THORACIC OUTLET
            SYNDROME
CAPSULITIS
TENNIS ELBOW
MEDIAN NERVE COMPRESSION
⎱ 6

MUSCULAR
    LOW BACK PAIN
SPONDYLOSIS
LUMBAGO
SCIATICA
ABDOMINAL
    HERNIAE
    CYSTOCELES
    VISCEROPTOSIS
    CONSTIPATION
ARTICULAR
    DISC
    LUMBO-SACRAL
VASCULAR
⎬ 4

BUTTOCK & HAMSTRING
    MUSCLE STRAIN
HIP JOINT INVOLVEMENT
⎱ 3

MUSCULAR
    PAIN IN MUSCLES OF
            FOOT AND LEG
    BUTTOCK & BACK PAIN
ARTICULAR
    JOINT PAIN (ANKLE, KNEE,
                    HIP)
    HALLUX VALGUS
    HALLUX RIGIDUS
PROLAPSE OF ANTERIOR
            TRANSVERSE ARCH
ANKLE AND FOOT STRAIN
STRESS FRACTURES
VARICOSE VEINS
⎱ 1

MUSCULAR
    TENDONS ON
    INNER SIDE OF
            KNEE
ARTICULAR
    MEDIAL COL-
    LATERAL LIGT.
    MEDIAL COM-
    PARTMENT
    OSTEOARTHRITIS
⎬ 2

FIG. 19
The effects of postural strain at the six fixing levels.

Knee joint

Muscular: Strain of the sartorius, gracilis and semitendinosus.

Joint: Strain on the medial collateral ligament and medial compartment of the joint. Osteoarthritis.

Vascular involvement: Varicose veins.

Hip joint

Muscular: Strain of the adductors and gluteii.

Joint: Strain of the joint structures generally causing a tight joint.

Lumbo-sacral

Muscular: 1. Direct: strain of muscles associated with the lumbo-sacral level.

2. Indirect: strain on the abdominal muscles due to pendulous belly and weight of abdominal contents. Herniae.

Joint: Lumbo-sacral disc involvement. Facet or apophyseal joint syndrome.

Nerve roots: True or pseudo sciatica.

Gastro-intestinal: Secondary effects from a protuberant abdomen, giving rise to a variety of gastro-intestinal symptoms, visceroptosis and constipation.

Head or neck

Muscular: Strain of the posterior cervical muscles.

Joint: Disc degeneration and osteoarthritis of the joints of Luschka and the apophyseal or facet joints.

Vascular: Involvement of the vertebral artery. Indirectly, cerebral symptoms. Headache, vertigo. Later, cerebral degeneration.

Nerve roots: Involvement of the cervical plexus. Neuritis, with pain in neck, shoulder girdle and upper arm.

Shoulder girdle

Muscular: Tenderness and spasm of the cervico-scapular muscles.

Joints: Capsulitis of the shoulder joint.

Vascular: Compression of venous and arterial circulation of upper extremities.

Nerve roots: Brachial neuritis.

Miscellaneous: Shoulder-hand syndrome. Median nerve compression.

This is a formidable list of effects. Some may consider the connection between them to be rather tenuous: but there is one factor which is common to all of them. They are invariably accompanied by a local upset in the circulation of the body fluids. The therapy we apply, therefore, must not only correct the mechanical derangement but also the local abnormality of the tissue fluids.

The treatment of such diverse conditions clearly varies considerable; but in the majority, rest, support, exercise, baths and massage will be needed. In all of them postural training is essential.

REFERENCE
GOLDTHWAIT, J. E. (1915). Anatomic and Mechanistic Conception of Disease. *Boston med. surg. J., 172,* 881-898.

CHAPTER VI

ACTIVE ALERTED POSTURE AND THE FOURTH CIRCULATION

The closed cardiovascular system consists of three circulations, the arterial, the venous and the lymphatic. However, there is another, a fourth circulation consisting of the fluid within cells composing the various tissues (intracellular fluid) and the fluid in the interstitial spaces between the cells (extracellular fluid).

Gamble (1947) has shown that 70 per cent of the body weight is made up of water, in which 5 per cent is in the plasma, 15 per cent is interstitial fluid. Fifty per cent is intracellular fluid (Fig. 20).

Franklin (1951), a prominent Harveian, gave a comprehensive description of the present views on the circulation. 'The blood circulation itself is but a part of the vast continuous movement of the body fluid as a whole, a movement by means of which even the cell constituents are constantly being removed and replaced so that no individual remains exactly the same from hour to hour or even minute to minute. The simple concept of the blood being pumped from the heart through the great arteries to the distant arterioles and capillaries, and then returning through venules and veins to the right auricle, has given way gradually to the realisation that a complete understanding of the circulation embraces the tissue fluid, lymphatic circulation and intra and extracellular changes'.

The tissue fluid circulation is composed of interstitial fluid and intracellular fluid, and I have called this The Fourth Circulation.

Naturally, the total volume of the circulation fluid depends on the intake and output of fluids, adjusted by the circulatory, renal and respiratory systems, with additional control exerted by the nervous system and the endocrine glands. The interchange of the

39

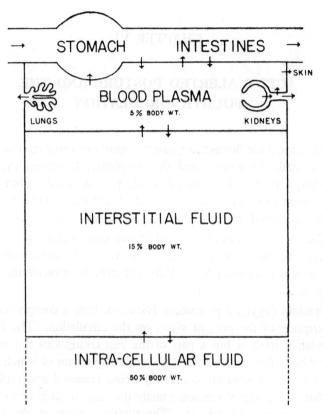

FIG. 20

Distribution of fluid in the body.

materials from the capillary to the cells by means of the interstitial fluid is determined by:

1. The barriers between them, i.e. the capillary and cell walls.
2. The effective hydrostatic pressure in the capillary.
3. The effective osmotic pressure.

The pumping action of the skeletal muscles is a most important factor in propelling the interstitial fluid, and helping in the interchange between the body cells and the interstitial fluid. If this pumping action of the muscles diminishes in any way, there is a tendency for oedema and deposition of metabolites in the tissues.

This is shown after a person who has been in bed for any length of time gets up and starts walking. There is a tendency for the ankles to swell, and the tissues to become tender to pressure. As the muscle tone is improved, or if massage is given with the limb in elevation, the swelling will gradually disappear, particularly if the dependant part is supported by an elastic bandage when the patient is upright.

It is interesting to conjecture why the tissues are tender. It would seem that they contain some chemical substance which causes tissue tenderness; and they remain tender as long as this substance is present in the tissues. Massage and exercise gradually disperse it, but as it spreads from the site of its original deposition to other tissue planes, these then become tender. Lewis called it the H substance. Other authorities consider it is one of the breakdown products of tissue metabolism, hyaluronidase or bradikinin. I call it the T substance, because it makes the tissues tender.

A similar condition of tissue tenderness occurs when a haematoma forms in the tissues as a result of a blow or injury. The haematoma spreads or seeps through the interstitial tissues of the muscles, areolar tissues and fascial planes, and this spreading or seeping of the haematoma is affected by gravity, the action of the muscles, the direction of the blood vessels, and configuration of the tissue planes. As this spread takes place to other parts, these tissues discolour, and take on a purplish, greenish, and yellowish hue. As the spread continues, so the tissues far remote from the original site of the injury become tender. This is probably due to haemosiderin in the blood pigment. However, until the haematoma is completely absorbed, this tissue tenderness remains, often far remote from the original site of injury.

One of the best ways of getting rid of haematoma is to aspirate it, or express it through an incision. If the haematoma has been present for some days, clots can be expressed, and sometimes the amount is of unexpected magnitude.

I maintain that there is another cause of stasis in the interstitial tissues – poor posture. What I describe as Inactive Slumping Posture is due to the unbalanced action of the muscles, so that there is just enough energy in the muscles on one side of the body to hold the body upright. In patients who are slumpers, the tissues become tender, particularly in relation to the antigravity muscles, and in my view this is due to the accumulation of the metabolites in the interstitial spaces of the muscles and areolar tissues, and is a result of the unbalanced action of the muscles in failing to get rid of them. So often, this tenderness of the tissues has been named fibrositis, or muscular rheumatism, conditions which many doctors consider do not exist, because nothing abnormal can be seen under an ordinary microscope. However, the muscles remain tender as long as these products are present. This tenderness will disappear with physical treatment and exercises in exactly the same way as a bruise, spreading and seeping through the tissues.

It seems to me that, if a person is a habitual slumper, or has unbalanced posture, the muscles are affected in this way right throughout life. Often the tissues become saturated with this chemical substance by the age of 30. In slumping posture, the muscles are not supporting the corresponding joints, and it becomes obvious that, in time, the joints will suffer strain. As soon as this happens, the muscles tend to go into spasm. Whenever a muscle is in spasm, its circulation is impeded and therefore more metabolites form. Eventually, due to joint strain and muscle spasm, the intra-articular structures, such as the articular cartilage and intervertebral discs – become involved, and osteoarthritic changes will appear. Of course, this is not the only cause of osteoarthritis; but it is an important one – because it is entirely preventable if **Active, Alerted Posture** takes the place of inactive, slumping posture. The muscles on each side of the body are then in slight balanced contraction. This constitutes a form of continuous isometric exercise, and the tissue fluids are being constantly circulated, with the disappearance of tissue tenderness.

REFERENCES

FRANKLIN, K. J. (1951). Aspects of the Circulation's Economy. *Br. med. J.* **1**, 1343-1349.
GAMBLE, J. L. (1947). *Chemical Anatomy, Physiology and Pathology of Extracellular Fluid.* 5th ed. Cambridge: Harvard University Press.

CHAPTER VII

INJURY: EFFECTS AND TREATMENT

In postural and occupational strain and the conditions which arise from them, there is a local upset in the circulation of the body fluids which must be corrected by treatment if the symptoms are not to be unnecessarily prolonged. There are even grosser fluid abnormalities to be found at the site of injury, where tissues may be so contused that they die, and where there may be extensive haemorrhage from ruptured vessels.

The body reacts to trauma exactly as it does to infection: the same inflammatory response occurs in both conditions. However efficient it may be at localising infection, the process is not an unmixed blessing at the site of an injury: the out-pouring of blood, and fluids with a high fibrin content, leads to the formation of adhesions between structures which normally should glide freely over one another. Moreover, when the fluids are especially abundant, as they often are where there is much dead tissue, they may delay healing considerably. This stage is sometimes called the 'negative' phase; and unless active measures are taken it may be prolonged and eventually result in dense adhesions. It is important, therefore, to disperse the excess fluids as quickly as possible.

If the condition is severe, as in direct trauma, operative treatment may be necessary: the dead tissue is excised, the blood clot and fibrin-rich serum expressed. The affected area can then pass into the 'positive' healing phase immediately, and with the minimum of adhesions. In less serious injury, where there is little dead tissue or haemorrhage, the swellings may be dispersed by physical means, for example firm massage after the injection of a local anaesthetic (10 ml. of Xylocaine with 1500 international units of hyaluronidase added to promote rapid dispersion) or surging faradism to the affected muscles.

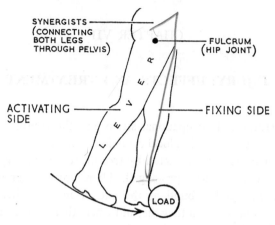

FIG. 21

This is a good example of balanced action in which the load (the ball) the force and the levers are as nearly as possible one above the other; also the activator leg must work with the assistance of synergists on the firm fixing leg.

Whether operative or physical dispersion has been used, the injured part needs firm support: but the support should be a removable one so that the patient can carry out the home treatment which will turn this positive phase into complete recovery.

There should be a certain degree of urgency in the treatment of all injuries, whether they occur in industry, in civilian life or in the athletic field. Of course, prevention is better than cure. Prevention of accidents is a complex but rewarding task. There are four main lines of approach.

1. Environmental precautions.

2. The security against unbalanced movement that comes from **Active Alerted Posture** (Fig. 21)

3. The understanding of the mechanics of movement, and, if an accident does occur, the analysis of the movement so that any faults may be corrected.

4. For athletes, basic training aimed at promoting general fitness. Examples are weight-lifting, power training, circuit training and yoga exercises.

To treat injuries, I recommend what I call the active therapeutic approach. This contains the following measures:

1. First aid treatment at the source of the injury.
2. Treatment at a medical centre, where a full diagnosis is made and specific therapy begun.
3. Home treatment by the patient.
4. Physiotherapy.
5. Occupational therapy: in a team this may be in the hands of the trainer.
6. Review by Rehabilitation Officer.

The types of home treatment are:
1. Rest from weight-bearing or strain (complete, moderate, minimal).
2. Exercises – these must be carefully graded.
3. Home massage.
4. Self manipulation.
5. Poultices.
6. Baths.
7. Support.
8. Medical.

This home treatment, which has the great advantage of continuity, is all important: but the additional attention of a skilled physiotherapist invariably accelerates recovery. Apart from the special measures he may employ, the physiotherapist is able to make certain that the patient is performing his exercises correctly and, where the back or lower limbs are affected, walking properly. The various types of physical treatment which may be given are heat (lamps, short wave), massage, faradic stimulation, manipulative therapy, anodal galvanism (sinusosoidal current), ultrasonic, interferential therapy, deep x-ray, ultra-violet ray and proprioceptive neuromuscular facilitation.

One special merit of properly designed physiotherapy is that the whole body can be maintained in condition while a special treatment is given to the injured part. This is reflected in the therapeutic approach at a famous football club – 'Treat and Train'. This active therapeutic approach accelerates the removal of necrotic tissue and inflammatory fluids, prevents adhesions, and by maintaining the length of the muscle fibres, prevents contractures. It also maintains and improves muscle tone and power, preventing the wasting so often associated with injury.

Muscle injury. Injuries to muscle may be classified as follows:
1. Those due to direct violence. The injury is a contusion.
2. Those due to indirect violence:
    (a) strains, including tear of a few fibres,
    (b) tear of a considerable number of fibres,
    (c) complete rupture,
    (d) tearing of the muscle with a large lump of bone, either at its origin or insertion,
    (e) traumatic tenovaginitis.

Joint injury. Injuries to joints may be similarly classified.
1. Those due to direct violence – contusion of the joint.
2. Those due to indirect violence:
    (a) a local tear of a few fibres of a ligament,
    (b) a moderate tear of a ligament with involvement of the synovial membrane or meniscus as shown by joint effusion,
    (c) Severe rupture of a ligament,
    (d) Rupture of a ligament with complications such as a fracture into the joint or involvement of the articular cartilage.

If a haematoma forms, every endeavour should be made to prevent any of several complications, shown in Figure 22.

Bone injury. Fractures may be caused by direct or indirect violence. They may even arise from sudden muscular contraction (for example, fracture of the patella) or from a trifling force because of some pathological condition like osteoporosis or a new growth.

If a fracture is stable, it needs only protection and support, which can sometimes be adequately provided by a bi-valve or split plaster. Such plasters have the great merit that they can be removed for home treatment and formal physiotherapy, to the great benefit of the patient; but even unstable fractures, held in position by plaster enclosure, traction or internal fixation, may

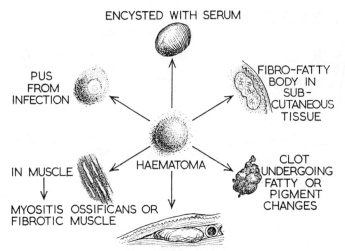

ENCYSTED WITH SERUM

PUS
FROM
INFECTION

FIBRO-FATTY
BODY IN
SUB-
CUTANEOUS
TISSUE

IN MUSCLE   HAEMATOMA

CLOT
UNDERGOING
FATTY OR
PIGMENT
CHANGES

MYOSITIS OSSIFICANS OR
FIBROTIC MUSCLE

PAINFUL THICKENINGS
a. WHERE CONVERGING TISSUE PLANES FORM "DEAD" AREA
b. NEAR MAIN BLOOD VESSELS

FIG. 22
Complications on haematoma.

be greatly benefited by home treatment, aimed at dispersing swelling, maintaining the tone and power of the muscles and preventing adhesions.

Where a limb is completely enclosed in plaster, postural drainage and isometric exercises can be carried out. It is even possible to give surging faradic contractions to the muscles through windows in the plaster (Fig. 23).

Trueta has shown how the pumping action of the muscles as carried out in isometric exercises or surging faradism stimulates the venous circulation, thus preventing stagnation of stale blood in the endosteal bone. This promotes callus formation and therefore the quick healing of fractures.

Plaster casts should be made to fit closely and snugly but should never feel tight or press on a bony point. Some padding over pressure areas is permissible. A plaster cast for a Colles' fracture should have the merit of allowing free movement of the

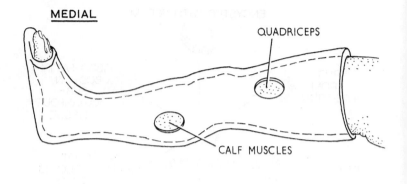

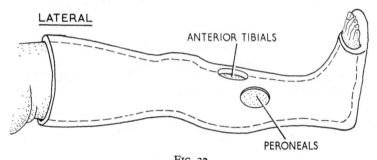

FIG. 23

Windows through the plaster of Paris at motor points so that surging faradism can be administered.

fingers and full spread of the palm as well as the elbow. To accomplish this the plaster should only reach as far as the first crease in the palm and just proximal to the knuckles of the hand below, at the same time reaching up to 2 inches below the bend of the elbow above (Fig. 24A).

In a plaster cast for a Pott's fracture the toes must be able to move freely; there must be plenty of breadth for the forefoot and the knee should be able to flex fully (Fig. 24B). Some orthopaedic surgeons advise a platform for the toes.

Traumatic syndromes: phases and stages. The process of healing cannot progress until all the traumatic swelling and dead tissues are removed. As soon as this negative phase finishes, the positive healing phase commences (Armstrong and Tucker).

The different phases and stages in recovery are well

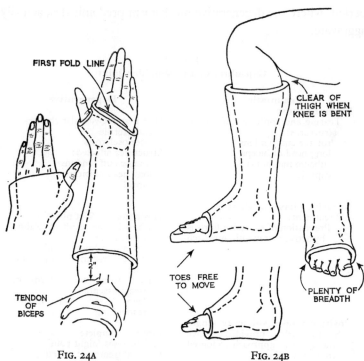

FIRST FOLD LINE

CLEAR OF
THIGH WHEN
KNEE IS BENT

TENDON
OF
BICEPS

2"

TOES FREE
TO MOVE

PLENTY OF
BREADTH

FIG. 24A
A type of plaster cast for
Colles' fracture.

FIG. 24B
Types of plaster cast for Pott's fracture.

demonstrated in the two main types of capsulitis of the shoulder, the first entirely due to injury, the second fundamentally due to vascular disturbances. Table I demonstrates the difference in the two conditions.

The progress of the degenerative type may be influenced by concomitant disease, as shown by a high sedimentation rate or a gouty diathesis; or by the presence of cervical spondylosis denoting disc degeneration and osteoarthritis, particularly of C5, 6 and 7.

Unfortunately, in some cases there is a combination of both injury and degeneration, and therefore in advising any form of treatment it is imperative to determine which stage and phase the condition has reached: for therapy which at one stage can be beneficial, whichever mechanism predominates, can at another

D

period, where the degenerative mechanism predominates, actually aggravate.

TABLE I

Capsulitis of the shoulder joint

Traumatic	Degenerative
Primary cause	
Tearing and contusion of certain structures:	Degenerative vascular changes:
rotator cuff tendons	endarteritis
long head of biceps	arteriosclerosis
subacromial bursa	Structures affected:
capsule	rotator cuff tendons
	long head of biceps
	capsule
Negative phase (acute stage)	
Treatment:	Girdlestone's 'Wet phase':
Prevention of excessive fibrosis by active therapeutic approach	Fibrosis, the result of healing incomplete
	Patient has 'night pain'
	Physical treatment may aggravate
	Rest from every form of strain essential
	Deep X-ray later, if not responding
Positive phase (subacute stage)	
Starts early, provided active therapeutic approach adopted from beginning	Fibrosis complete
	Patient loses 'night pain'
	Physical treatment effective
Chronic stage	
Entirely avoidable by proper treatment	Not entirely avoidable but susceptible to modification in terms of time to recover

REFERENCE

ARMSTRONG, J. R. & TUCKER, W. E. (1964). *Injury in Sport.* p. 291 London: Staples Press.

CHAPTER VIII

OSTEOARTHRITIS AND HOME TREATMENT

Fundamentally osteoarthritis is a wearing away or flaking off of the articular cartilage of the opposing surfaces of a joint. The cartilage cells pile up on the periphery and form osteophytes.

Signs and symptoms vary, but some grossly involved joints may manifest few symptoms. The first thing a patient may notice is a little joint stiffness, accompanied by a rheumatic ache in the surrounding muscles. The only sign may be a slight limitation of movement. The radiograph is often normal.

It is at this stage that the disease can be checked. The problem is one of early diagnosis, since many patients do not report what they regard as the trivial muscular rheumatism to be expected in middle age. Yet, just as mass chest radiography has helped to control tuberculosis, so, if the joint movements of all persons over forty years old were checked at intervals of a few years, we could detect limitation of movement often denoting early osteoarthritis at a time when it would still respond to a combination of home treatment, physiotherapy, manipulation and injections. At this stage, with careful treatment, there may be regeneration of articular cartilage and substantial recovery of the joint; but even when the patient becomes symptom-free, he is well advised to continue home treatment conscientiously and indefinitely, in order to guard against future relapses.

Osteoarthritis has been divided by many authorities into:

1. primary, idiopathic and

2. secondary, due to some predisposing factor.

I maintain, as many people do, that except in the case of osteoarthritis affecting several joints of the hands and wrists at middle age, especially in women, that most cases of osteoarthritis should be considered as secondary: and the primary factors to which it is secondary are as follows.

(a) *Damage of soft tissues and bony structures* by severe or repeated small injuries. A lumbar disc or knee injury can leave the thigh muscles weak or contracted, with effects on the hip joint. Injured joints, especially weight-bearing ones, must be restored to full range of movement and muscle power whenever possible.

(b) *Inactive slumping posture*, adopted by most people throughout life. This produces muscle strain, which, in time, progresses to joint strain and later osteoarthritis, especially in weight-bearing joints.

(c) *Dysplasia*, from congenital causes, affecting soft tissues and bony surfaces, such as occurs in congenital subluxation of the hip.

(d) *Incongruity of the acetabulum and the head of the femur* as occurs in Perthes' disease and slipping of the femoral epiphysis.

(e) Activation of articular cartilage degeneration by endocrine (androgen and oestrogen) imbalance around the age of fifty. This may be the associated cause in primary osteoarthritis affecting many joints of the hand and wrist.

(f) *Thrombosis of a segmental artery* to the femoral head; aseptic necrosis of a section of the femoral head (D'Aubigne *et al.*, 1965).

In osteoarthritis, from whatever cause, there may be a 'tight joint', that is to say a joint in which there is limitation of the normal average range of movement. The tightness of the joint structure may result from congenital tight muscles, capsule, and other soft tissue around a joint; or it may be the result of muscle spasm due to involvement of the joint. All treatment should be directed to overcoming joint tightness.

Some chemical substance which forms in the osteoarthritis process is undoubtedly responsible for the tissue tenderness. Just as the tissue tenderness from injury is thought to be due to haemosiderin, so in osteoarthritis, Lewis's H substance, hyaluronidase, or bradykinin may be the cause. I call them collectively the 'T' substance, the characteristics of which are that it causes tissue tenderness and that it behaves, when being absorbed, like a bruise, spreading and seeping through the tissue. As other signs and symptoms disappear, so this tissue tenderness gets less and less.

Exacerbations and painful episodes may be due to a number of possible causes.

1. The patient may have put the joint to excessive use or used it in some new way by a change of exercise or occupation.

2. He may have stretched adhesions by forced movement of a restricted joint. These adhesions may have formed as a result of protective muscle spasm with contraction of the capsule.

3. There may be a septic or toxic focus. Gout is not the cause of osteoarthritis but an osteoarthritic joint may be subject to an attack of gout.

4. A small piece of articular cartilage may have separated. Pain and general aggravation of symptoms will persist until the raw area has healed over or the small piece has become enveloped by the synovial membrane. At operation, an osteoarthritic hip may contain hundreds of small pieces of articular cartilage which have gradually become extruded and enveloped by the synovia. They appear like bunches of grapes suspended around the joint periphery, each one possibly representing an attack of pain and increased stiffness.

5. There may be a subluxation of the joint due to alteration in the weight-bearing surface. This may be sudden or gradual, but in either case the symptoms are usually acute.

6. A synovial fringe or villus may have been nipped, with consequent haemarthrosis.

In all cases there is tenderness of the tissues around the joint and often, until movements and muscle power return to normal, symptoms will continue.

The treatment of osteoarthritis may be considered under the following headings.

Preventive measures

There are three main types of strain against which preventive measures should be taken.

TABLE II

Types of strain	Prophylaxis
Postural	Active alerted posture
Occupational	Improved mechanical tools and working environment
Excess weight	Weight reduction
A further important measure is the care of joints previously injured	

General treatment

TABLE III

The general assessment of the patient

The search for and elimination of septic or toxic foci

The search for and treatment of gout

Exact instructions as to the correct amount of rest and exercise

Specific anti-rheumatic medicines

Analgesics

Local treatment

Category 1. Home Treatment with periodic courses of physiotherapy.

Category 2. Home Treatment with periodic courses of physiotherapy; and hydrocortisone or other injection therapy.

Category 3. Home Treatment with intra-osseous injections, manipulation under pentothal, deep X-ray Therapy.

Category 4. Home Treatment with minor operations – tenotomies, myelectomies, local arthrotomies, joint irradiation by Cobalt 60 Needles.

Category 5. Home Treatment with major operations (Figs. 25 and 26).

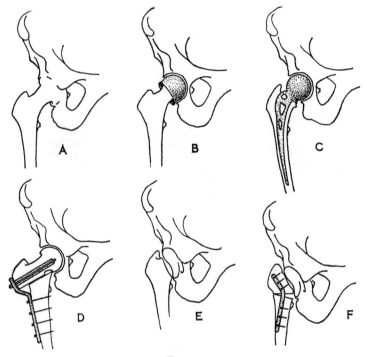

FIG. 25

Various types of major procedures.

A. Arthrodesis; B. Smith Petersen cup arthroplasty; C. Austin Moore arthroplasty; D. McMurray's osteotomy with internal fixation; E. Girldestone's exision of the femoral head; F. Batchelor's modification of Girldestone's procedure with osteotomy and internal fixation.

Operations are indicated because the patient fails to improve after four months of intensive conservative treatment. It may be that:

1. night pain persists or worsens,

2. the patient becomes less mobile,

3. deformity of the limb increases or

4. where the patient is relatively young, he may need an operation in order to carry on with his required activities.

There is a particular operation suitable to almost every case in which operation is indicated. The hip is the joint for which operation is most often required, and the major hip operations are:

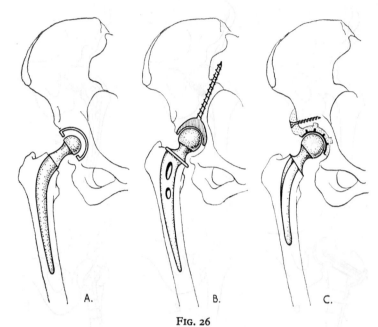

FIG. 26
Total Hip Replacement.
A. Charnley; B. Ring's; C. McKee Farrar.

Muscle and capsular release. Decompression of the joint by muscle and capsular release as in the Voss operation, the 'hanging hip'. It is essential to release the adductor muscles, gluteus medius and minimus, attached to the greater trochanter, and 'Forage' or drilling of the neck and head must be included. In my own practice, I release the adductors by open operation above, at the same time tenotomising the tendon of insertion of adductor magnus just above the adductor tubercle on the inner side of the knee joint. The rectus femoris is also released, and a good section of the anterior capsule is removed. The greater trochanter is released by osteotomy and a forage carried out. This is a good operation in very early cases where a high degree of efficiency is required in a young patient. It can carry him over a period of activity necessary for his particular requirements. It is also applicable to the aged, as it is an operation that can be accomplished in 20 minutes: it can therefore be tried before more drastic measures are undertaken.

Osteotomies. Adjustment of the lines of strain as in MacMurray's displacement osteotomy of the femur with internal fixation. This also tends to decompress the joint (Fig. 25D).

Arthrodesis. A good operation on one side in joints destroyed by injury and subsequent osteoarthritis in relatively young patients (Fig. 25A).

Arthroplasty. These operations both decompress the joint and remove the products of the osteoarthritic process on one or both sides of the joint.

(a) Smith Petersen cup arthroplasty (Fig. 25B).

(b) Austin Moore or Thompson vitallium/prosthesis arthroplasty (Fig. 25C).

(c) An endoprosthesis with both an acetabular and femoral stem elements:

    1. The Charnley type (Fig. 26A.)
    2. The McKee Farrar type (Fig. 26C).
    3. The Ring type (Fig. 26B).
    4. The Stanmore type.

Removal of arthritic bone. Removal of the arthritic femoral head as in Girdlestone's operation (Fig. 25E) or Blount's and Batchelor's pseudo-arthrosis (Fig. 25F). Similar operations may be carried out in other joints, for example the removal of the patella for patello-femoral arthritis, the trapezium for osteoarthritis of the carpus and the outer end of the clavicle for painful osteoarthritis of the acromio-clavicular joint.

Operation on nerves, spinal cord or brain stem. For relief of pain. This form of therapy is now seldom employed.

Even after a successful operation, home treatment must be continued. The corresponding joint on the opposite side, and those above and below, must be included; that is to say, in osteoarthritis of the right hip, the right knee, the low back and the left hip must all be included in the daily routine exercises.

The osteoarthritic patient must realise that there is no cure for his condition; but if he is prepared to devote half an hour twice each day to home treatment, he may keep himself free of pain and reasonably mobile for a long time. Operation need be advised only when the prescribed home treatment is not holding the osteoarthritic process in check.

REFERENCES

d'AUBIGNE, M., POSTEL, M., MAZALSAND, A., MASSIAS, P. & GUEGUEN, J. (1965). Idiopathic necrosis of the femoral head. *J. Bone Jt Surg.* **47-B**, 612-633.

CHARNLEY, J. (1968). Total prosthetic replacement of the hip. *Sandoz J. med. Sci.* **8**, 211-216.

McKEE, G. K. & WATSON-FARRAR, J. (1966). Replacement of arthritic hips by the McKee-Farrar prosthesis. *J. Bone Jt. Surg.* **48-B**, 245-259.

RING, P. A. (1967). Total hip replacement. *Proc. R. Soc. Med.* **60**, 281-284.

VOSS, C. (1956). *Munch. med. Wschr.* **98**, 954-956.

CHAPTER IX

MANIPULATIVE TREATMENT

Just a hundred years ago, Sir James Paget (1867) wrote in the *British Medical Journal* an article entitled 'Cases the bone setter cures'. Before and after this period, many qualified medical men as well as unqualified manipulators, have obtained good results following sound manipulative techniques.

Sir Robert Jones taught that, in a joint disabled by injury or certain diseases, the degree of limitation of movement should never be ascribed to functional causes until the effects of manipulation under an anaesthetic have been tried. A joint with limited movement, especially if painful, is bound to deteriorate unless the range of movements and the muscle power have been restored to as nearly normal as possible.

Every practitioner, if he follows the fundamental principles of manipulation, as laid down by Mennell (1949), can develop simple manipulative techniques, which are safe and can accomplish good results in suitable cases. Mennell's technique was based upon three fundamental principles:

1. The extensibility and flexibility of joint structures should be restored by traction and countertraction (Fig. 27).

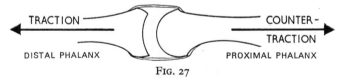

TRACTION — COUNTER-TRACTION

DISTAL PHALANX   PROXIMAL PHALANX

FIG. 27

First Principle of Manipulation applied to Phalanges.
Traction and Countertraction.
This helps to restore the extensibility and flexibility of the soft tissues.

2. While these separating forces are applied, the accessory involuntary movements which restore the gliding, rotatory, and sliding movements of one bone on another are executed (Figs. 28, 29 and 30).

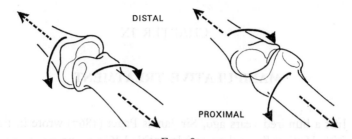

DISTAL

PROXIMAL

FIG. 28

Second Principle of Manipulation.
Traction and Countertraction with rotation of one phalanx on another. This helps to restore joint play movements or the involuntary movements of the joint.

3. Still under traction and countertraction, the range of active movement up to the point of pain is carried out, with the difference that in flexing the joint, the distal part is helped in flexion, whereas the proximal part is pressed in the opposite direction (Fig. 31).

In the small joints, such as the finger and wrist, the manipulator can apply traction and countertraction by distracting the articular surfaces of the joint by the use of both hands. However, in the larger joints he may require an assistant to carry out the countertraction (Fig. 32).

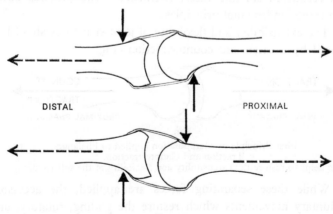

DISTAL   PROXIMAL

FIG. 29

Traction and Countertraction. The distal phalanx is moved forwards and backwards.

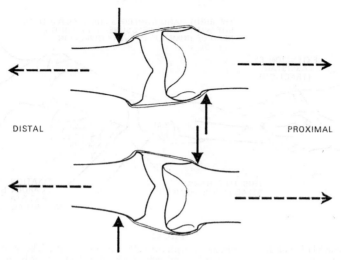

FIG. 30

Traction and Countertraction. The distal phalanx is moved sideways in both directions on the proximal.

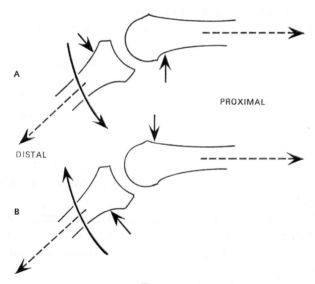

FIG. 31

Third Principle of Manipulation applied to Phalanges.
This helps to restore full active movements.

A. Flexion of distal phalanx on proximal.
B. Extension of distal phalanx on proximal.

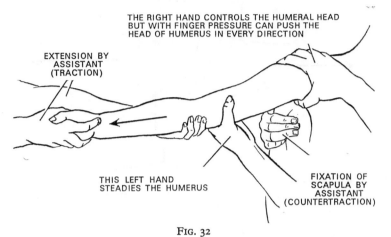

THE RIGHT HAND CONTROLS THE HUMERAL HEAD
BUT WITH FINGER PRESSURE CAN PUSH THE
HEAD OF HUMERUS IN EVERY DIRECTION

EXTENSION BY
ASSISTANT
(TRACTION)

THIS LEFT HAND
STEADIES THE HUMERUS

FIXATION OF
SCAPULA BY
ASSISTANT
(COUNTERTRACTION)

Fig. 32

Manipulation of the Right humerus with the help of two assistants. The humeral head can be pushed downwards, forwards, backwards and upwards in the glenoid fossa. The use of long lever action must be avoided.

Certain rules for manipulation must be strictly followed.

1. An exact diagnosis must be made.

2. The phase or stage through which the condition is passing must be established.

3. Any septic or toxic focus must be eliminated before manipulation.

4. The reaction to manipulation must be expected to be moderate – that is to say, the patient should be expected to recover from this reaction within 48 hours.

5. As certain muscles act through more than one joint, the joint above and below must also be put through a full range of movement i.e. in the case of the knee, the movements of both hip and ankle must be restored to normal.

6. No undue force must be applied. Gentle handling of the tissues must be carried out, employing the use of a short lever; and movements must be of low intensity, though sometimes of high velocity.

7. First class ancillary treatment must be combined with the manipulative movements: home treatment, postural training, rest, intermittent traction, removable support, exercises, injection therapy and other forms of physiotherapy.

8. Manipulation under an anaesthetic, if indicated, should be left to the specialist in this field.

In restoring full movement, both voluntary and involuntary, there must be gradual improvement each day. If improvement ceases, the patient's condition should be carefully checked and, if necessary, further investigated. A period of rest may be desirable; or, if gross adhesions or internal derangements are thought to be causing the limitation of movement, manipulation under anaesthesia may be considered.

There is a wide field for manipulation. The principal objects are:

1. To eliminate muscle spasm and restore full movement, the involuntary accessory movements as well as the voluntary active movements. Where any muscle has been torn, manipulation helps to restore full extensibility and flexibility to the injured muscle.

2. To adjust intra-articular structures such as the menisci of the knee.

3. To adjust subluxations, such as occur in the facet or apophyseal and tibiotaloid joints.

In many cases, the patient himself can be taught simple self-manipulative movements, and this technique is described in Instruction number 17 of Part 2, page 112.

The principal conditions for which manipulation is prescribed are as follows.

1. Recent injuries.

2. Postural, occupational and recreational strain.

3. Osteoarthritis.

4. Capsulitis of the shoulder joint, or 'frozen shoulder' (Table I Chap. VII).

5. Backache. Of course, this is a symptom, and can occur as a result of injury, postural strain and osteoarthritis, and other previous conditions; but it should be considered as an entity itself.

6. Miscellaneous group, including Rheumatoid arthritis.

REFERENCES
MENNEL, J. B. (1949). *The Science and Art of Joint Manipulation*. London: Churchill.
PAGET, Sir JAMES (1867). Cases the bone setter cures. *Br. med. J.*, **1**, 1-4.

CHAPTER X

BACK ACHE

Pain in the back frequently begins because the muscles do not support the underlying vertebral joints. There may have been a severe injury or a sudden twist; or the patient may have been sitting in a draught. Whatever the reason, the muscles fail to take the strain, and the joint, being unsupported, becomes painful. The joint lesion may prove to be a simple sprain, but in the lumbar and cervical regions, an intervertabral disc is often affected, either by compression, disintegration, or protusion.

In an occasional patient, there may have been a slipping of one vertebra upon another (spondylolisthesis). In all cases of persistent back pain, therefore, it is advisable to take several views when x-raying the lumbar spine. In addition to the usual A.P. and lateral views there should be oblique and lateral views with the spine in flexion and extension. If there is evidence of spondylolisthesis, in-patient hospital treatment may be needed.

To prevent recurrence of strain, the patient must learn to assist the lumbo-sacral vertebral joints, by the active, protective, supporting action of the muscles. At first this may not be possible, because the muscles have been made weak and atonic. A period of inaction is therefore indicated. He may have to have absolute rest in bed; this will certainly be required if the pain tends to radiate down either leg, especially if there is pain on coughing, sneezing or bending. If he cannot possibly rest in bed, the next best thing is a plaster jacket or rigid corset (Fig. 33) which will rest the back but let him get about (ambulatory rest). As soon as the pain has gone, he must practise isometric exercises in the jacket to strengthen the muscles.

In mild cases, where there is no evidence of sciatica, physiotherapy (including gentle manipulations) may help to adjust joint derangements of the posterior or apophyseal joints and

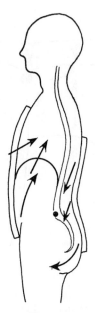

FIG. 33

Ambulatory rest in plaster of Paris. This allows the patient to walk about but helps to fix and rest the lumbo-sacral level by the plaster support and the balanced contraction of the abdominal, back and buttock muscles.

restore muscle tone. As the patient's symptoms pass off, remedial exercises are helpful, but must often be combined with firm support of the lower back. For the rest of his life, the patient must remain 'low back conscious', and guard the lumbo-sacral joints, locking them in a safe position by the active, balanced contractions of the abdominal, buttock, and erector spinae muscles. This is achieved by pelvic tilting: the abdominal muscles are held up and the buttocks are tucked under and made hard, as if one were leaning on a shooting stick. Thus, when the patient bends, lifts, coughs, sneezes or makes any trunk movement which might cause strain, the abdominal, buttock and back muscles are contracted in unison, the lumbo-sacral junction is firmly fixed, and the risk of displacing an intervertebral disc or producing subluxation of an apophyseal joint much reduced (Fig. 34). He must learn never to perform any sudden movement

E

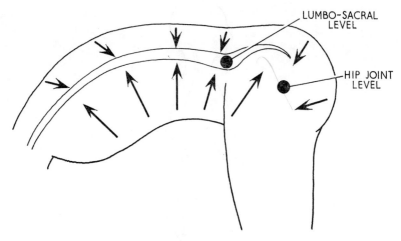

FIG. 34
Bending so that the action takes through the hip joint as the pivot point. The abdominal muscles actively pull down the truck and are in balance with the back and buttock muscles so that there is no strain on the lumbo-sacral level. The joints at this level are locked and fixed by the balanced action of all muscle groups.

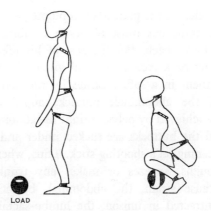

FIG. 35
The right way to lift; load, force and lever are as near as possible one above the other. The lumbo-sacral level is firmly fixed.

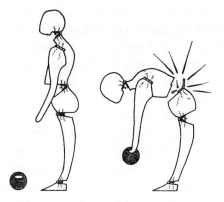

FIG. 36

The wrong way to lift resulting in an unstable lumbo-sacral level.

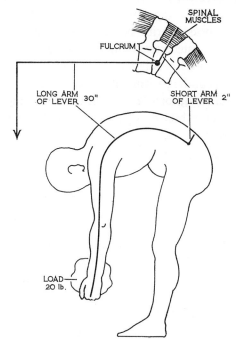

FIG. 37

If 20 lb. is lifted 30 in. away, the momentum of force working on the lumbo-sacral disc is 15 × 20 + weight of arms + weight of head and trunk, i.e. about 400 lb. in men and 350 lb. in women.

of the trunk, upper extremities and head unless the prime fixors at the junction of the trunk with the pelvis are firmly contracted (Fig. 35). Only if he forgets, or is taken off his guard, is he likely to do further damage. Moreover, he must not attempt to lift at a mechanical disadvantage, for the strain is enormous (Figs. 36 and 37).

In the last 30 years, the general public has been made over familiar with the diagnosis 'slipped disc'. There is a tendency to assume that all cases of back pain are due to involvement of the intervertebral disc: but, in fact, the symptoms may be due in the first place to strain of the muscles, and only later to involvement of the joint structures, of which the intervertebral disc is the most vulnerable. The final stage is spondylosis, in which there is not only disc involvement but osteoarthritis as well. If the posterior or apophyseal facets (apophyseal joint) of the vertebrae are involved in the osteoarthritic process, and sometimes when there is no evidence of osteoarthritis, they may become locked, in the same way as a drawer gets jammed. This causes severe pain.

The prognosis of the patient with backache is not easy to assess: if he has a prolapsed, torn disc, or an unstable joint, it may only be possible to cure him by operation: but the majority, if they conscientiously carry out home treatment, especially the home massage and baths, if they do their exercises regularly and pay full attention to posture, have a good chance of staying symptom-free for years.

CHAPTER XI

SUGGESTIONS ON THE CONDUCT OF HOME TREATMENT

Printed instructions to describe simple actions very often have a formidable appearance. It may take a page of words to describe an action which can be performed in a second. It is very natural, therefore, for a patient to be dismayed when he is handed a series of instructions on home treatment, and to wonder how he can get through all the items in a day.One of the objects of the series is to save the doctor time and trouble, and yet ensure that the patient has all the necessary instructions for his treatment. But, if they are to succeed in both purposes, they do not absolve the doctor from all trouble. It is essential for him to spend a few minutes discussing the instructions with the patient; and he should advise how the treatment may be fitted in to the patient's day.

Obviously if the patient has suffered an injury and is not able to carry on his normal life, he will have more time to carry out home treatment and he should set aside three periods of half an hour and four other periods of 5 minutes for treatment – not a great deal in 24 hours. During the half-hour periods, say from 8 to 8.30 a.m., 2 to 2.30 p.m. and 8 to 8.30 p.m., he should perform the contrast bathing, the home massage and the special exercises. During the evening period he should perhaps substitute a hot bath for the contrast bathing.

If the patient is to carry out baths, exercises and other forms of home treatment, it is obvious that any support must be of a removable type. During the periods of rest, some type of poultice may be considered helpful.

At 10 a.m., noon, 4 p.m. and 6 p.m. he should practise the special exercises for 5 minutes.

As recovery progresses he can take more and more exercise with increasing strain.

A patient can become expert in giving himself the proper massage – gentle stroking at first, but as the condition becomes more chronic, deep friction and kneading will become possible. If there is an injury at the front of the elbow or over the quadriceps, he must be warned of the dangers of the formation of bone in the soft tissue structures.

In chronic conditions like osteoarthritis, so long as symptoms are present the patient is well advised to carry out home treatment conscientiously twice a day for half an hour. If the condition is getting worse, he may feel that he is fighting a losing battle; but it is disastrous to give up, because the deterioration is sure to accelerate. At this stage he should consult a doctor again and even consider an appropriate operation.

If the symptoms settle and the patient becomes relatively symptom free, home treatment once daily for half an hour may be sufficient to prevent the recurrence of symptoms.

Neither the home treatment nor the contributory measures such as dieting, postural drainage and the practice of **'Active Alerted Posture'** require much physical effort, but they do need determination. If the patient can be made to realise that he owes a duty to himself, that only by his own efforts can he keep himself as fit and well as his age and the condition of his tissues allow; if he can be persuaded to take an active instead of a passive attitude to his health, he will persevere even in the most chronic disease. Only his doctor can give him the initial determination and the constant support he needs; but the reward will be great for both doctor and patient. To save a patient from joining the ranks of querulous and hopeless chronics is not only good medicine: it is a service to the whole community.

PART II

Instructions for Patients

INSTRUCTION 1

REASONS FOR HOME TREATMENT

For many reasons, the muscles and soft tissues may become contracted and lose their resilience and suppleness. This has a marked detrimental effect on their extensibility and flexibility, and therefore on the movements of the joints involved. Also, gradually the joints themselves undergo strain, which leads to degeneration. Home treatment can help to ward off:

1. the effects of postural, occupational and recreational strain,
2. the effects of injury,
3. the effects of degeneration,
4. the effects of infection and
5. the effects of the general ageing of the tissues.

Try to adopt a sensible attitude towards home treatment from the start, because if you do practise it regularly you may prevent your condition from getting worse or avoid possible complications. There are a number of things you can do at home, and your doctor will tell you which of them he wants you to do and how to do them.

1. Active Alerted Posture

The first thing you have to learn and practise is how to stand properly—a way of standing called **Active Alerted Posture.** Once you have learnt this you need fewer special exercises, because when you stand correctly, you are exercising your muscles constantly.

2. Rest

The painful part may need rest and support in the position your doctor shows you.

73

3. Massage

While you are in the bath, massage the painful part with soap. After the bath, massage it with powder, oil or cream.

4. Baths

The doctor will tell you if he wants you to have frequent baths in the ordinary sense of the word, or whether he wants you merely to bathe the injured part. Baths to the injured part may be hot, or what are called 'contrast baths' – alternate hot and cold baths or sponging.

5. Exercises

You may have to do some simple exercises several times a day, or twice a day after bathing the injured part. Do these exercises without straining or causing pain.

6. Poultices

The doctor will tell you if he wants you to apply poultices and when.

7. Physiotherapy

Do not confuse this with the physiotherapy they give you at hospital. This is physiotherapy you give yourself at home, such as heat from lamps, or electrical treatment to make the muscles work. You must be careful to follow your doctor's instructions exactly.

8. Postural drainage

This phrase means putting the injured part in such a position that the fluid will drain away from it and the swelling will go down.

9. Common sense

Use your common sense. Don't sit in draughts or work in unfavourable conditions, or do anything unwise.

INSTRUCTION 2

THE PROPER WAY TO STAND

Have you ever thought how many times you move your muscles and joints in a year? If they are going to keep doing their job, year after year, they should be used in the most efficient way.

Your muscles have two functions: first they fix and lock the joint, as when you are standing still: second they move the joint.

Now think of a movement of the arm – say a backhand stroke at tennis (Fig. 2, 1). The muscles of the hand and forearm make the movement. They are helped by other muscles at the wrist, elbow and shoulder: but the whole movement depends upon the fixing of the shoulder girdle, to give the arms something solid

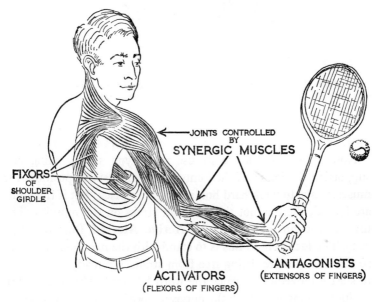

FIG. 2, 1

To demonstrate how the correctly executed backhand tennis shot is performed by activators acting in conjunction with synergists and prime fixors.

75

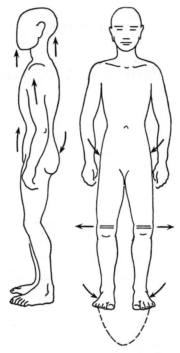

Fig. 2, 2

Active Alerted Posture is also balanced, concentric posture. Muscles on opposite sides of the body are in slight isometric contraction.

to move on. You can see that, in any movement, the job of some muscles is to produce movement, but of others to fix and lock.

Now your muscles are in use when you stand, fixing and supporting the joints. If the joints are in an unstable position, the muscles have to work hard holding them in place; but if the joints are locked, there is not this constant strain on the muscles. The first instruction told you about **Active Alerted Posture** (Fig. **2, 2**). The idea behind this is to stand with the main joints locked, so that the muscles, being free from strain, are ready at any time to start a movement – hence the word 'alerted'. This is the ideal position. Compare it with the opposite position you see in slovenly people – the Inactive Slumping Posture (Fig. **2**, 3). They look tired, and they are tired; because the weight of their limbs, head

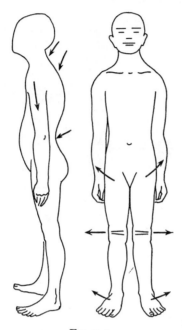

FIG. 2, 3

Inactive Slumping Posture is also imbalanced, eccentric posture. Gravity strains are not prevented.

and trunk, is dragging on the muscles, causing continual strain on the ligaments and other joint structures. You must avoid this posture at all times because it is bad for the muscles and bad for the joints. If you stand correctly, in the way you are told in the next section, your body cannot feel the weight of the head, the limbs or the trunk.

Lifting and loosening the shoulders counteracts the pull of the weight of the arms and helps to support the head. By tucking in the buttocks and tilting the pelvis forward the internal organs are supported. Bending the knees slightly gives the cushioning effect of a spring. Arching the instep and gripping with the toes takes the weight off the innerside of your feet and stops them going flat.

TOP OF HEAD TRYING TO TOUCH THE CEILING

SHOULDERS LIFTED AND
HELD SLIGHTLY FORWARD

NAVEL PRESS-BUTTONED
TO SPINE

BUTTOCKS
PINCH-PROOF

KNEES
SLIGHTLY BENT

GROUND GRIPPED
WITH TOES

WEIGHT ON OUTER SIDE OF FEET

FIG. 2, 4

This illustrates the various positions of the body in perfect Active Alerted
Posture.

How to acquire an Active Alerted Posture

(Fig. 2, 4)

1. Pull up the arch muscles of the foot so that the weight is
carried evenly on the heel and the outer border, the forefoot
gripping the floor with the toes, knees slightly bent.
2. Tilt the pelvis so that the stomach muscles are held up and
contracted, with the buttocks tucked under and the buttock
muscles firmly contracted. Stand as if you were balanced on a
shooting stick.
3. The shoulders should be slightly up, the chin tucked in, and
the head balanced on the shoulders so that there is no tendency

for the head to fall forwards. The effect of this is to make the back of the neck as long as possible and fix the shoulder girdle firmly to the chest wall.

This is Active Alerted Dynamic Posture in preparation for action

1. *Ankles and feet:* Stand like a successful bow-legged jockey, not like a knock-kneed, flat-footed tramp.
2. *Low back and hips:* Stand with a rock-bottom and pinch-proof posterior instead of sag back with prominent belly.
3. *Head and shoulder girdle:* Stand as if the top of your head were linked to a star, instead of with the rounded, sloping shoulders of a beggar.

INSTRUCTION 3

GENERAL ADVICE TO PATIENTS

Your doctor will tell you which of this list of home treatment measures he wants you to adopt.

1. Rest from strain.

    You may walk – not at all
         a little
         a moderate amount
         as much as you like
    You may lift – not at all
         a little
         a moderate amount
         as much as you like

2. Support.
    Belt, bandage, plastic splint, plaster splint, strapping, sticks, crutches.

3. Exercises.
    (a) General. See Instructions 6-15
    (b) Yoga. See Instruction 17

4. Postural Training.

5. Postural Drainage.

6. Baths. The doctor will explain to you what to do.
    (a) Contrast showers or baths
    (b) Hot baths, hot sponging

7. Home Physiotherapy.
    (a) Heat lamp
    (b) Wax baths
    (c) Electrical treatment (Faradism)
    (d) Massage

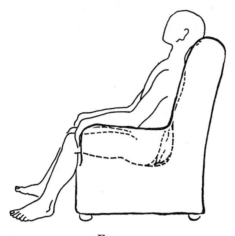

FIG. 3, 1

Passive Supported Posture; sitting with the joints in neutral position.

8. Poultices.

(a) Antiphlogistine or Kaolin at night three times weekly

Method of application. Warm the tin of Antiphlogistine or Kaolin for 2 minutes in hot water; spread some on to a piece of lint as if you were buttering bread; cover with a piece of gauze to prevent it sticking to the skin; heat before a fire or on a saucer over a pan of boiling water; test against the arm before applying; cover with cotton wool, oilskin and bandage. A ready-prepared poultice (Medilintex) may be used instead.

(b) Liquor hammamelis

(c) Lead and opium

(d) Hot towel compresses

9. Diet.

This is to reduce your weight. See Instruction 20

10. Preventive Treatment.

You can do a good deal to avoid further trouble.

(a) Always use **Active Alerted Posture** when you are standing or in any position when you are going to move.

(b) Don't work in an uncomfortable position. Try to get the job arranged so that you can work without getting cramped.

(c) If you have back trouble, sleep on a hard bed with the pillows arranged as follows: four pillows in an inverted A: one

F

pillow represents each arm of the A and two are placed across the top: the head is thus supported in the neutral position (Fig. 3, 1, 2, 3).

    (d) Avoid draughts.

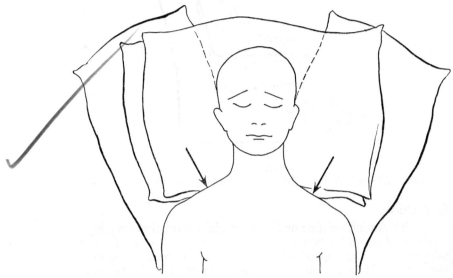

FIG. 3, 2
Passive Supported Posture; lying – front view.

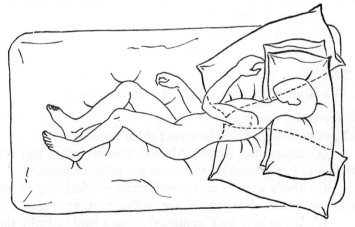

FIG. 3, 3
Passive Supported Posture; side view lying with the joints in neutral position.

INSTRUCTION 4

GENERAL RULES FOR EXERCISES

Exercises are best done when the joints have been warmed up by soaking in a hot bath, by radiant or infra-red heat lamps, before a coal, electric or gas fire, or by taking contrast baths.

Do each movement slowly and deliberately. When you have moved the part as far as you can in one direction, try to coax it a little bit further – but do not jerk it or force it.

The sequence of graded exercises is as follows.

1. Without weight-bearing or strain:
   - (a) With the aid of gravity
   - (b) With the aid of a sling
   - (c) Exercises in water

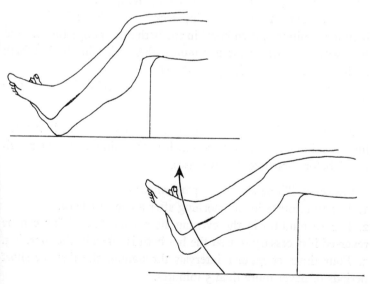

FIG. 4, 1

The right ankle and foot cross over the left ankle and foot; resistance to straightening the left knee is made by the right leg.

2. With strain:
    (a) Against gravity
    (b) With graduated weights
    (c) Against strong resistance (Fig. 4, 1)
3. Weight-bearing exercises:
    (a) Gentle
    (b) Moderate
    (c) Strenuous

Contrast baths. This means soaking the part to be exercised in hot water for 2 minutes, then in cold water for 2 minutes. Go on doing this for 10 minutes. Start with hot and finish with hot, thus:

Hot	*Cold*	*Hot*	*Cold*	*Hot*	*Total*
2 mins.	2 mins.	2 mins.	2 mins.	2 mins.	10 mins.

    (a) A spray or shower is the best method, as it can be used hot or cold on any part of the body (Figs. 4, 2 and 4, 4).

    (b) For a limb: if you have no shower or spray, use two basins of water, one hot and one cold (Fig. 4, 6).

    (c) For the back or hip, neck or shoulder: lie in a hot bath for 2 minutes, then kneel in the bath and sponge the affected part with cold water for 2 minutes, then relax in the hot bath again for 2 minutes (Fig. 4, 5). Repeat.

    (d) Ice. Rub the painful area with ice cubes held in a face cloth (Fig. 4, 3).

At the end of your hot bath, cool the water so that it is tepid for one minute before you get out. Rub the skin well with a rough towel before starting the exercises.

Exercise. These should be performed:
1. For 10 minutes in the morning after a contrast bath.
2. For 10 minutes in the evening after a hot bath. This can be reversed if necessary so that the hot bath is taken in the morning.
3. Four times at regular intervals throughout the day for short periods of never more than 5 minutes.
The rhythm of the exercise is important. Do it by numbers until you get the rhythm.

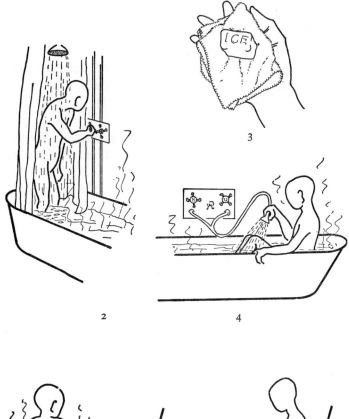

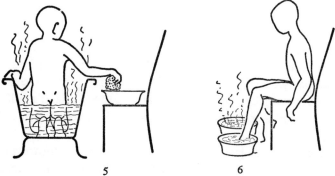

FIG. 4, 2-6
Different ways of taking contrast baths.

1. Tighten the muscle.
2. Keep it tight.
3. Let the muscle go.
4. Relax.

You must not overdo it. If the part swells or becomes stiff, the exercises have probably been too vigorous. Do not exercise when you are tired – but be careful not to make this an excuse for not exercising.

As your condition improves, you should increase the number of exercises you do each time. Start off by performing each exercise six times, but you may increase this figure quite rapidly. If you really want to get well you must do the exercises religiously, regularly and resolutely.

If you are young and have been injured in a strenuous sport, like professional football, and are trying to get fully fit to get back to your sport, the exercises illustrated in this book can often be stepped up rapidly. Of course, all swelling and painful movement of the injured part must have disappeared before you attempt vigorous exercises. They should include those of your basic training:

1. Weight-assisted exercises. Power training.
2. Interval training exercises.
3. Circuit training.

The exercises illustrated in the instructions should each be carried out slowly six times at first, increasing the speed, and number gradually as recovery occurs. They can also be carried out 'isometrically', that is to say against resistance, which can be your own resistance – for example resisting the left hand's pull by the right hand – or that of some assistant for 7 seconds each exercise.

The exercises suggested and listed in the various instructions may be carried out in combination for certain conditions, such as back pain, forms of tennis elbow or osteoarthritis of the various joints. If you carry out all the exercises suggested for a particular joint, every muscle connected with that joint is exercised.

INSTRUCTION 5

REACTION TO HOME TREATMENT

It is sometimes possible to get some ill effects after home treatment. You may have increased swelling, stiffness, tenderness or pain in the damaged muscles and joints.

This instruction explains why, and tells you what to do.

There are two likely reasons for the ill effects: first, you may have some unsuspected condition, like a tendency to gout or some hidden infection: second, and more likely, you may have made too energetic a start on your treatment.

If the reaction follows a Turkish bath, you may have stayed in too long or been too vigorous with massage and manipulation after the bath. On the next occasion, reduce the time of the bath – half an hour is quite long enough at the start – gradually increasing it with each treatment: and be more gentle with your massage and manipulation.

If the reaction follows exercises, reduce the time you spend on them by half and increase it by a minute each day up to a maximum of fifteen minutes' exercise and fifteen minutes' massage twice a day.

Pain and stiffness after weight-lifting exercises may be a sign that the joint is not yet ready for these exercises. If you are certain that you have used only the weight specified by your doctor, give up the exercises until you have consulted him.

Slight reaction to home treatment is to be expected, especially if the muscles are sore before you start: and if you persevere, the soreness will soon wear off. A certain amount of discomfort, including some pain, must be tolerated in restoring full function to damaged muscles and joints. If, on the day after a rather strenuous session of home treatment, there is increased swelling and pain, it is best to continue more gently until the condition has settled. You may find that you have improved, in spite of the temporary apparent set-back.

Remember the golden rule: if in doubt, consult your doctor.

INSTRUCTION 6

PAIN IN THE ARMS, SHOULDERS, NECK, BACK AND LEGS

Pain in the shoulder and arm

Pain in the shoulder may be due to trouble in the neck, and pain in the arm and hand to trouble in the neck or shoulder. But sometimes, the elbow or the shoulder becomes painful because of some condition lower in the arm. It is always best, therefore, to exercise the arm and shoulder as a whole, from wrist to neck. Exercises in Instructions 7-12 must all be carried out.

Pain in the neck or back

Your backbone, which stretches from your head to your tail, consists of a number of vertebrae separated by flat plates of gristle called discs. The vertebrae are supported and controlled by muscles. Pain in the neck or back may be due to a strain of the muscles, or of a group of vertebrae.

The little discs between the vertebrae sometimes become damaged if you move suddenly at a time when the muscles supporting the vertebrae are slack. This is most likely to happen in the neck or the lower back, because these are the places you move most. With the pain there is usually stiffness, which may be so bad that the part becomes rigid.

If the pain is not very severe, the condition may be treated by physiotherapy and gentle manipulation. If it is very severe, or if it does not react to this treatment, you may have to go to bed for a complete rest, and, when you get up, wear a support for your neck or back. In either case, to complete the cure and to avoid another attack, you must learn how to fix the joints in your neck and back, whenever you are going to move. You do this by performing exercises and by learning **Active Alerted Posture.**

Until your symptoms have completely gone, you must keep

your spine absolutely rigid. If you want to pick up something you must bend your knees and hips, *not* your back. For some time you must not lift anything heavy, and when the doctor allows you to lift again, you must make sure, in order to lessen the strain, that anything heavy is very near you.

If you have any stiffness in the neck, shoulder girdle or shoulder, this will throw more strain on the low back; thus if there is trouble in the low back, it is essential to have resilience of the neck, shoulder girdle and shoulder joint muscles. So you should invariably exercise the whole lot – shoulder, shoulder girdle, neck, back, hips, knees, ankles and feet. Exercises in Instructions 10-16 must be carried out.

After severe back strain, there is always a tendency for the spine to stiffen and get painful as you grow older. Daily home massage, baths and exercises will help to delay this tendency, perhaps for a very long time, perhaps for ever.

Pain in the legs, including the buttocks and hips

Pain in the buttocks, hips, thighs and legs may be due to trouble in the back: and pain in the lower back may be due to trouble at one of the joints below. So it is as well to treat the whole area as one, and you should do all the exercises for the lower part of the body, from the waist down, as in Instructions 13-16. This ensures that there will be balanced action of all the muscles – of the back, buttocks and legs.

INSTRUCTION 7

FINGERS AND HANDS

This group of exercises is designed to put the joints through their full range of movements and at the same time strengthen the associated muscles.

(See General Rules for Exercises, Instruction 4)

1. Make a clenched fist, squeezing on a bandage or ball of wool. (Fig. 7, 1).
2. Strum on a table or a desk as if you were playing a piano. (Fig. 7, 2).
3. With your palms flat on a table, spread your fingers apart and bring them together again. (Fig. 7, 3).
4. With your palms flat on a table, lift your fingers separately off the table, so as to extend each finger; (Fig. 7, 4a) then lift all your fingers together, extending the tips backward. (Fig. 7, 4b).
5. Touch the tip of each finger with the tip of your thumb. (Fig. 7, 5).
6. Bend your fingers at the knuckle joints at the same time straightening them at the finger joints, as in the writing position. (Fig. 7, 6).

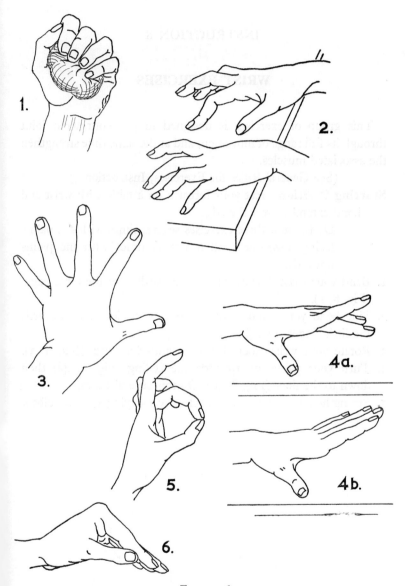

FIG. 7, 1-6

Finger exercises.

INSTRUCTION 8

WRIST EXERCISES

This group of exercises is designed to put your wrist joint through its full range of movement and at the same time strengthen the associated muscles.

(See General Rules for Exercises, Instruction 4)

Starting Position – rest your forearm on a table with wrist and hand extended over the edge.

Do the first three exercises several times with the palms facing downwards, then several times with the palms upwards.

1. Bend your wrist downwards and upwards over the table edge. (Fig. **8**, 1).
2. Side bend your hand towards the thumb side, then towards the little finger side. (Fig. **8**, 2).
3. Rotate your wrist clockwise, then anti-clockwise. (Fig. **8**, 3).
4. Turn your palms up towards the ceiling (Fig. **8**, 4a) then down to the floor (Fig. **8**, 4b). Do this several times.)
5. Strengthen your forearm muscles by carrying out the elbow exercises.

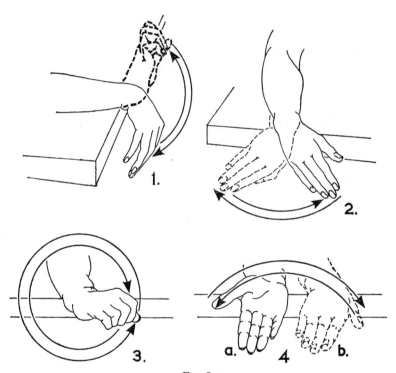

FIG. 8, 1-4
Wrist exercises.

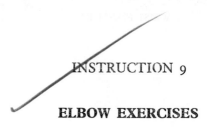

INSTRUCTION 9

ELBOW EXERCISES

This group of exercises is designed to put the elbow joint through its full range of movement and at the same time strengthen the associated muscles.

(See General Rules for Exercises, Instruction 4)

The first four exercises are done with an unopened roll of bandage held in the hand.

A. *Starting position* – arms at side. (Fig. 9, 1a)

  1. Palms facing forward, squeeze the bandage as you bend the elbow (Fig. 9, 1b). Return to the starting position, relaxing the pressure on the bandage as you straighten the elbow. Squeeze bandage on bending; relax on straightening.

  2. Repeat the exercise with the palms facing backwards. Squeeze bandage on bending; relax on straightening. (Fig. 9, 2a and 2b).

B. *Starting position* – elbows bent.

  3. Palms forward (Fig. 9, 3a), straighten the forearm, squeezing the bandage (Fig. 9, 3b). Return to the starting position, relaxing the squeeze as you bend the elbow. Squeeze bandage on straightening; relax on bending.

  4. Repeat the exercise with the palms facing backwards (Fig. 9, 4a and 4b). Squeeze bandage on straightening; relax on bending.

  5. Do an imaginary tennis back-hand shot, but hold the upper arm with your free hand, so that the movement is nearly all made at the elbow. (Fig. 9, 5).

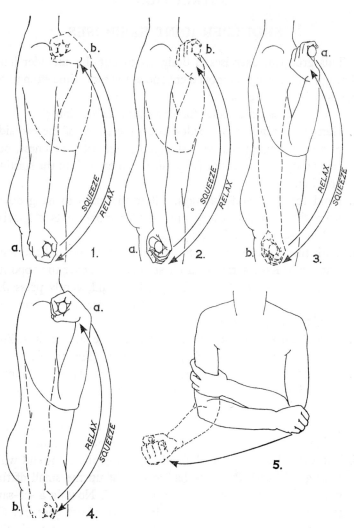

FIG. 9, 1-5
Elbow exercises.

INSTRUCTION 10

SHOULDER JOINT EXERCISES

This group of exercises is designed to put the shoulder joint through its full range of movement and at the same time strengthen the associated muscles.

(See General Rules for Exercises, Instruction 4)

1. Hang your arms at your sides. Bend the elbow of the bad side to a right angle (Fig. **10, 1a**). Keep it against your chest, but carry the *forearm* outside (Fig. **10**, 1b), then back to the starting position.

2. Bend forwards and sideways. Allow the arms to hang down from the shoulder. Carry out circular movements clockwise and anti-clockwise. (Fig. **10**, 2).

3. With the tips of your fingers touching your body all the way, bring your hand across your chest until it lies over the opposite shoulder (Fig. **10**, 3a). With the other hand, gently press the elbow of the limb being exercised towards the opposite shoulder (Fig. **10**, 3b).

4. Lock the hands behind the head, bracing the elbows back. You can do this standing or lying on your back (Fig. **10, 4**).

5. Starting position: lie down on your back with the fingers intertwined across the front of the body (Fig. **10**, 5a), lift the bad arm with the good arm until the hands are above the head (Fig. **10**, 5b). Return to the starting position, carrying the weight of the bad arm by the hand of the normal arm.

6. Put a towel over the good shoulder. Grasp the front end with your good hand. Push the bad arm right up the small of the back and grasp the other end of the towel. Now do a see-saw movement as though you were drying your back (Fig. **10**, 6).
   Note 1. This last exercise will not be given you until the shoulder is recovering. In the early stages, it may make the shoulder painful and stiff.
   Note 2. Some of these exercises can be done with the weight of the arm taken by a sling, or held by another person.

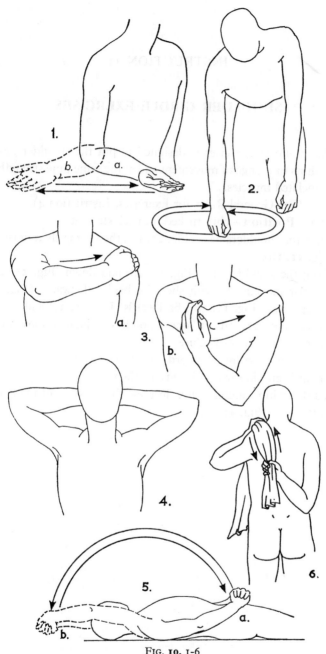

FIG. 10, 1-6
Shoulder exercises.

G

INSTRUCTION 11

SHOULDER GIRDLE EXERCISES

This group of exercises is designed to put the shoulder girdle through its full range of movement and at the same time strengthen the associated muscles.

(See General Rules for Exercises, Instruction 4)

Starting Position – chin tucked in, neck straight.

1. Brace the shoulders back (Fig. **11**, 1a), then bring them forward (Fig. **11**, 1b).
2. Shrug the shoulders up (Fig. **11**, 2a) and down (Fig. **11**, 2b).
3. Circular movements with shoulder blades, forwards (Fig. **11**, 3a) upwards (Fig. **11**, 3b), backwards (Fig. **11**, 3c) and downwards (Fig. **11**, 3d) in one smooth continuous movement. Then reverse the procedure.
4. Place hands, palms forward on desk, table or wall, press forwards and inwards (Fig. **11**, 4), then relax.
5. Hands on hips, increase and decrease the pressure of the hands on the hips (Fig. **11**, 5).

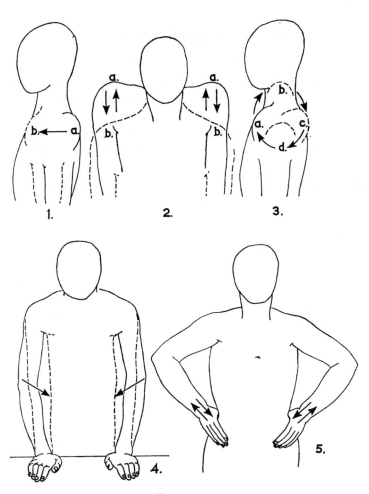

FIG. **11**, 1-5
Shoulder girdle exercises.

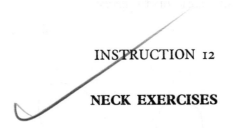

INSTRUCTION 12

NECK EXERCISES

This group of exercises is designed to put the joints through their full range of movement and at the same time strengthen the associated muscles.

(See General Rules for Exercises, Instruction 4)

Starting Position – Sitting in chair or lying down on couch or floor, chin tucked in, neck straight (Fig. **12**, 1a).

1. Bend your head forwards (Fig. **12**, 1b) and then backwards (Fig. **12**, 1c).
2. Turn your head to the right (Fig. **12**, 2a) and then to the left (Fig. **12**, 2b).
3. Sit on a chair and grip the edge of the seat with your hands. Side-bend the head as if to touch the ear on to the shoulder, first to the right (Fig. **12**, 3a) and then to the left (Fig. **12**, 3b). Do not raise the shoulders.
4. Rotate your head clockwise and then anti-clockwise (Fig. **12**, 4).

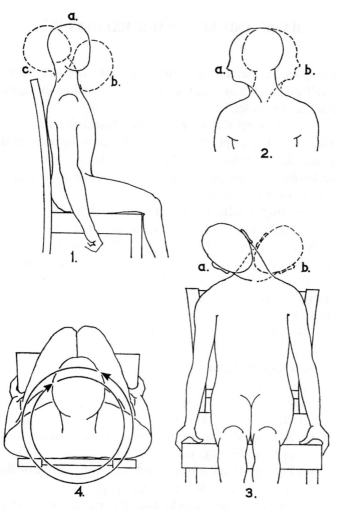

Fig. 12, 1-4
Neck exercises.

INSTRUCTION 13

BACK AND LOW BACK EXERCISES

This group of exercises is designed to put the joints through their full range of movement and at the same time strengthen the associated muscles.

(See General Rules for Exercises, Instruction 4)

A. These exercises employ muscles which attach the trunk to the pelvis and the pelvis to the thigh. They teach you to stand with the abdominal muscles pulled up and the buttocks tucked under so that the back is flattened.

1. **Starting Position** – lie on your back with your legs straight and the heels about 6″ from the wall.

   With your shoulders still, and keeping both heels on the ground with the feet at a right angle, try to stretch the left leg to touch the wall. Relax, then do the same with the right. In this exercise first one leg is made longer, then the other, and vice versa.

   The pelvis is tilted first to the left and then to the right (Fig. **13**, 1).

2. **Starting Position** – lie on your back (with knees bent) on the floor or on a couch (Fig. **13**, 2a).

   Raise your head off couch or floor and then relax back to the starting position (Fig. **13**, 2b).

3. (a) Arch your back, keeping your buttocks on the couch or floor (Fig. **13**, 3a).

   (b) Press your spine downwards on to the couch or floor so as to flatten the back (Fig. **13**, 3b).

   (c) Tighten your buttocks together, raising them off the couch or floor, keeping the feet and back firmly on the couch or floor (Fig. **13**, 3c).

B. The next four exercises are designed to strengthen the group of muscles producing movement at the waistline.

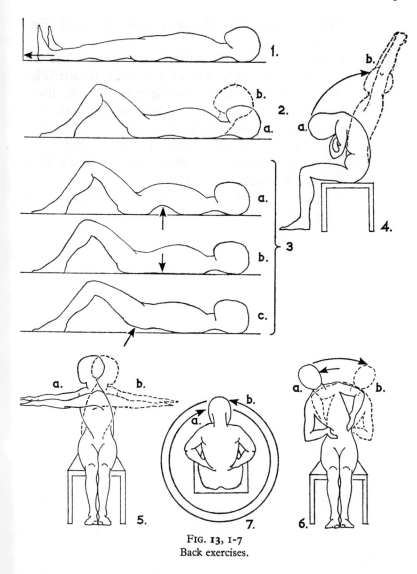

FIG. **13**, 1-7
Back exercises.

Starting Position – sit on a chair or stool with your legs
firmly fixed on the floor.
4. Bend your back forwards, breathing out with arms folded
across your chest (Fig. **13**, 4a). Straighten your back,

breathing in, raising the arms above the head (Fig. **13**, 4b).

5. Sit with your arms held out in front of you. Rotate the trunk first to the right (Fig. **13**, 5a), then to the left, (Fig. **13**, 5b), with the arms swinging parallel to the floor.

6. Hands on hips, side-bend to the right (Fig. **13**, 6a), straighten, and then side-bend to the left (Fig. **13**, 6b).

7. Hands on hips, combine all these movements by:

   (a) bending, rotating and side-bending the trunk in a clockwise direction (Fig. **13**, 7a).

   (b) repeating the same movements in an anti-clockwise direction (Fig. **13**, 7b).

NOTES

INSTRUCTION 14

HIP EXERCISES

This group of exercises is designed to put the hip joint through its full range of movement and at the same time strengthen the associated muscles.

(See General Rules for Exercises, Instruction 4)

Starting Position – lie on back.

1. Brace your knees straight with the feet slightly apart and rotate your hips by turning the toes inwards (Fig. **14**, 1a) and outwards (Fig. **14**, 1b).

2. Bend one knee to the chest and carry out circular movements clockwise and anti-clockwise (Fig. **14**, 2).

3. Raise your leg with knee straight, up, out, across and down to the starting position (Fig. **14**, 3a, b, c).

If you find exercises 2 and 3 too difficult, leave them out and do 4 instead.

4. Lift up your knees as high as you can, with your heel remaining on the bed. Allow the leg to fall first outwards, then inwards (Fig. **14**, 4).

Starting Position – lying on the side of the good hip.

5. Raise the affected leg sideways with the knee straight, then move the whole leg backwards (Fig. **14**, 5a, b).

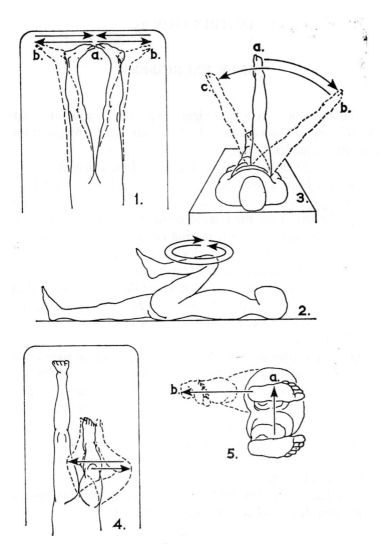

FIG. 14, 1-5
Hip exercises.

INSTRUCTION 15

KNEE EXERCISES

This group of exercises is designed to put the knee joint through its full range of movement and at the same time strengthen the associated muscles.

(See General Rules for Exercises, Instruction 4)

1. Sit upright on a couch with your legs stretched out straight in front (Fig. 15, 1a). Tighten the thigh muscles by straightening the knee from the relaxed position (Fig. 15, 1b). Do this as a slow, deliberate act, bracing the knee back hard. Count two and then relax the muscles completely. This exercise can be performed several times a day so that it becomes a habit.
2. Starting from the same position, brace the knee straight, then lift the whole leg upwards (Fig. 15, 2a), outwards (Fig. 15, 2b), across (Fig. 15, 2c), and then back to the resting position (Fig. 15, 2d).
3. Sit on the edge of a couch with a cushion under your knees and your legs hanging down (Figs. 15, 3a). Straighten one knee firmly (Fig. 15, 3b). At the same time bend the other knee, pulling the calf hard against the resistance of the couch (Fig. 15, 3c). Slowly and deliberately change position so that the bent knee becomes straight, and vice versa.
4. Lie on your back, hips and knees bent, and do bicycling movements with legs.

Patients with low back pain or elderly patients should perform this exercise with caution (Fig. 15, 4).

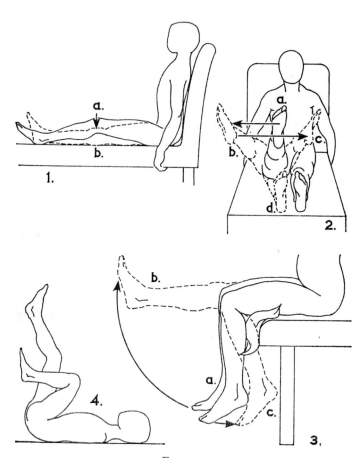

FIG. **15**, 1-4
Knee exercises.

INSTRUCTION 16

ANKLE JOINT, FEET AND TOE EXERCISES

This group of exercises is designed to put the joints through their full range of movement and at the same time strengthen the associated muscles.

(See General Rules for Exercises, Instruction 4)

1. Carry out circular movements of the feet clockwise and anti-clockwise. Keep the knees braced back and the legs still (Fig. **16**, 1).
2. Turn the soles inwards to face each other, then turn them outwards (Fig. **16**, 2).
3. Bend the feet backwards so that the toes are upwards (Fig. **16**, 3a), then downwards so that the toes point downwards, then relax (Fig. **16**, 3b).
4. With the forefoot supported so that the base of the toes is resting against something hard, such as a bed rail or edge of a board, bend the toes, keeping the toe joints straight (Fig. **16**, 4a). Then splay the toes and extend them (Fig. **16**, 4b).

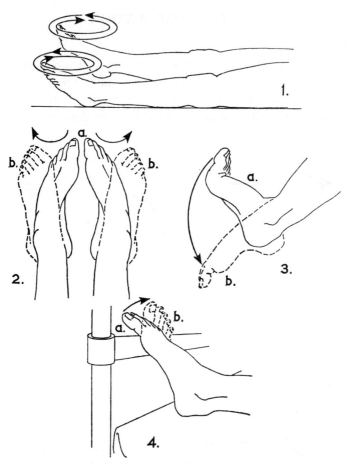

FIG. **16**, 1-4
Ankle, tarsal and metatarsal exercises.

INSTRUCTION 17

SELF MANIPULATION

In some joints, you can yourself carry out the main manoeuvres of manipulation – but only if your doctor advises it.

1. You can stretch your finger joints, by exerting a direct pull on the end of a finger against the resistance of the hand and wrist (Fig. **17**, 1).

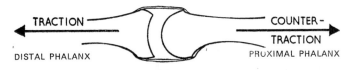

FIG. **17**, I

First Principle of Manipulation applied to Phalanges.
Traction and Countertraction.
This helps to restore the extensibility and flexibility of the soft tissues.

2. Maintaining this steady pull, carefully twist the finger and bend it from side to side (Fig. **17**, 2). Do not hurt yourself.

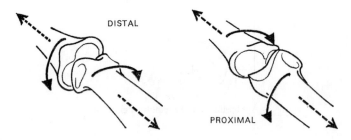

FIG. **17**, 2

Second Principle of Manipulation.
Traction and Countertraction with rotation of one phlanx on another. This helps to restore joint play movements or the involuntary movements of the joint.

3. Maintaining the steady pull, allow the finger to bend itself, stretch again in the direction it normally moves (Fig. 17, 3). Again, do not hurt yourself.

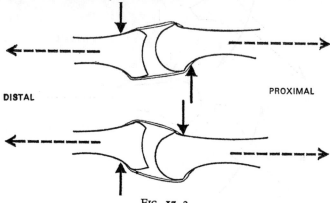

DISTAL   PROXIMAL

FIG. 17, 3

Traction and Countertraction.   The distal phalanx is moved sideways in one direction.

These exercises are best done in a hot bath, or immediately after a hot bath, when the muscles and sinews are warm. Other joints may be manipulated in a similar fashion (Figs. 17, 4 to 17, 9).

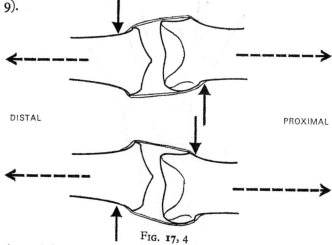

DISTAL   PROXIMAL

FIG. 17, 4

Traction and Countertraction.   The distal phalanx is moved sideways in both directions on the proximal.

H

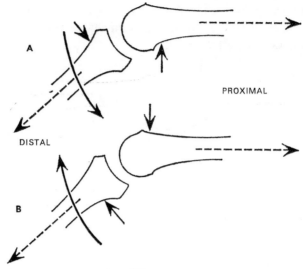

FIG. **17,** 5

Third Principle of Manipulation applied to Phalanges.
This helps to restore full active movements.

A. Flexion of distal phalanx on proximal.
B. Extension of distal phalanx on proximal.

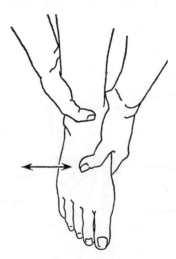

FIG. **17,** 6

The right ankle is fixed with the right hand and the left hand moves the foot
inwards and outwards. This helps to free the ankle and middle joints of the foot.

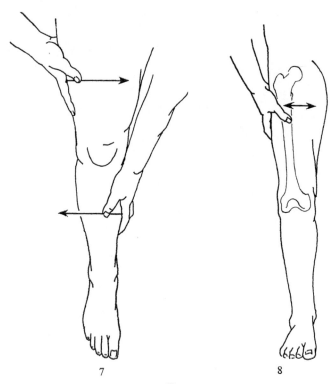

7   8

FIG. **17**, 7

The thigh is pushed inwards, the lower leg outwards. This manoeuvre opens
up the inner side of the knee.

FIG. **17**, 8

The upper part of the shaft of the right femur is shaken inwards and outwards.
This has the effect of a slight movement of the femoral head in the acetabulum
(hip socket).

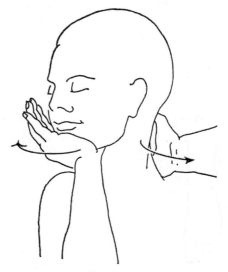

FIG. **17,** 9

Rotation of the neck to the right is assisted by the right hand twisting the chin
to the right and the left hand twisting the neck to the left. This helps to mobilize
the axis on the atlas, i.e. the second cervical vertebra on the first.

NOTES

INSTRUCTION 18

YOGA EXERCISES

These exercises are meant to make you supple, so that your joints can move through their full range. They are basically stretching exercises, and should be performed slowly and gradually, until you have reached the point beyond which you can no longer stretch comfortably. Stop whenever the movement becomes difficult or painful: there must never be any question of strain. Hold the position for a few seconds at first, then gradually longer each time. The aim is to increase the stretching and the time you can maintain it – but always without undue strain.

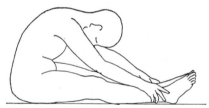

Fig. **18,** 1

Sitting on the floor, bend upwards and grasp shins as near the ankles as possible; pull downwards, and allow elbows to bend outwards.
This stretches neck, back, thighs and calves, also shoulder girdles.

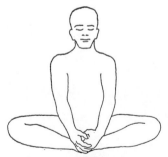

18, 2

Sit upright, flex and spread knees. Place soles of feet together and pull up to thighs with fingers of both hand intertwined.
This stretches the front and inside muscles of thighs as well as soft-tissue structures of knees.

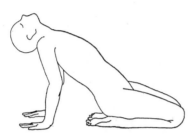

FIG. **18,** 3

Sit on ankles and bend trunk and head backwards with toes pointing downwards
and backwards.
This stretches soft tissues of ankles, knees, hips, back and neck.

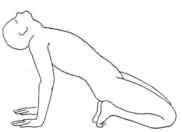

FIG. **18,** 4

The same exercise with toes up.

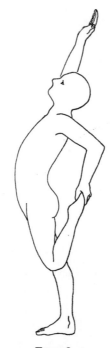

FIG. 18, 5

The left leg is grasped with the left hand, and the right arm is stretched up. In order to balance, lean the right thigh against a table or side of the bed. Turn round, and do the exercise using the opposite limbs.
This exercise stretches the quadriceps fully, and hyperextends the hip joint

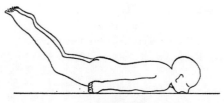

FIG. 18, 6

Lying face downwards, with fists pressed firmly on the floor, lift the legs backwards.

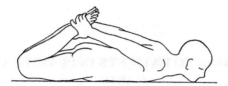

FIG. **18,** 7

Lying face downwards, bend the knees, and grasp the feet.

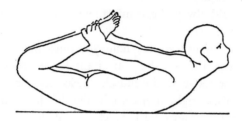

FIG. **18,** 8

Raise the head, pulling on the legs to extent the spine and hips fully.

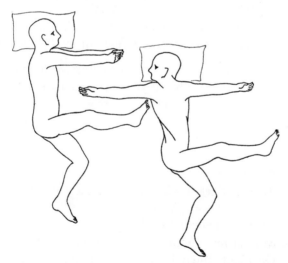

FIG. **18,** 9	FIG. **18,** 10
Lie on the left side, with the right leg over the left, and the arms stretched to the left.	Twist the head, trunk and right arm slowly to the right and hold.

This exercise has the effect of placing a twisting movement at the lumbo-sacral level.

INSTRUCTIONS TO PATIENTS IN PLASTER OF PARIS CASTS

If you have to wear a plaster case, it is most important for you to know what to do.

1. It should always be comfortable and should not squeeze or press you.
2. For two minutes *every* hour you must move your fingers or toes, holding the arm or the leg up above you. Try also to move all the muscles inside the plaster: you will feel them tighten against it. Do this many times a day.
3. The plaster must be kept clean and dry. You must tell your doctor, or go back to hospital, AT ONCE if:
   (*a*) The plaster cast is painful or presses on you.
   (*b*) The fingers or toes feel numb.
   (*c*) The fingers or toes become swollen or discoloured.
   (*d*) The fingers or toes become stiff and difficult to move.

At the start you may be allowed to walk with crutches but without putting any weight on your bad leg. Later you may be allowed to put some weight on the leg, though it is still in plaster.

This is the way to walk with crutches or sticks. You can do it to the count of three, or the count of four (Fig. **19**.)

The count of three:
  One. Crutches forward about 12 in.
  Two. Bad leg forward (in the air, if you are not allowed to put weight on it).
  Three. Swing the good leg through.

The count of four: Some people find this easier.
  One. Left crutch forward about 12 in.
  Two. Right foot forward in line with the crutch.
  Three. Right crutch forward.
  Four. Left foot forward in line.

Don't put either crutch too far forward – not more than 12 in.

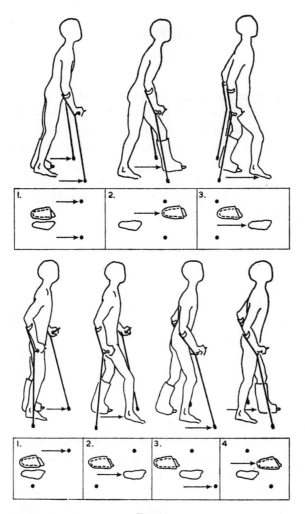

FIG. 19

SLIMMING

By Molly Castle

In this diet-conscious age everyone knows what calories are:
the measure of the amount of heat or energy released by the
combustion of food in the body. You can't eat a calorie any more
than you can eat your bathroom scales – but both measure all too
accurately just how much you do eat. If, during a day you consume
the amount of food which measures 2500 calories, you have to
use up exactly that amount of energy to remain at a constant
weight. Should you eat less, you will lose; more, and you will
gain.

Some people burn their food faster than others; they may take
in 4000 calories a day and still remain slim. Their inner furnace,
or metabolism, may be speeded up, or they may really use up the
energy. These are the people who never seem to relax or sit still,
and often they need to take less sleep than the quieter, lazier
ones. Some burn food very slowly, their metabolism rate is low
and their energy output likewise. These may gain weight on 1500
calories. They do not use up as much as they take in and the excess
is stored as fat. These lazy, relaxed ones often blame their glands,
their heredity or their worries for their overweight. These are
alibis but not good ones because, as Dr John Yudkin, Professor
of Nutrition and Dietetics says: 'Glands, worry, food habits may
make you eat too much in relation to your needs, but none of
these, all by themselves, gets some fat out of thin air, and whilst
you aren't looking, sticks it to your hips or tummy or wherever.'

Slimming experts differ on reducing methods, though all agree
that in to-day's civilised world we eat too much high carbohydrate
(over-processed, devitalised sugar and flour products) either for
figure or health.

In recent years some successful diets have been based on this very fact. It has been discovered by many experts in the nutrition world – among these, Professor Yudkin, as well as many American and European specialists – that it is the calories from carbohydrates rather than those from protein and even fat that cause excess weight.

I know this is an unpopular theory – most people hope for some magic pill – but the only sound way to get slim and remain so is to retrain your appetite so that you no longer like the nutritionally deficient, fat-producing pies, puddings and pastries. A taste for all food except milk is, after all, gradually acquired. Eskimos enjoy blubber, cannibals relish a plump missionary and man went along for several million years without a single lump of sugar. You can get all the carbohydrates you need from fresh fruit and vegetables, or natural sugars such as honey, which also supply needed vitamins and minerals removed from processed white sugar and white flour. True, bakers claim that white flour is 'enriched'. That is, quite a few vitamins and some minerals are put back after a good many more have been removed. And I very much doubt if these same bakers would consider themselves 'enriched' if someone stole £24 from them and then gave them back five or six.

So, instead of high carbohydrates eat plenty of protein (meat, fish, eggs, cheese, milk or milk products are the best sources, though nuts, whole grains and vegetables supply a certain amount). It is from the protein reserve that the body's repair work is carried out and protein supplies the bricks for this repair. If there is no protein reserve available the resourceful body will use any old bric-a-brac it can find in the blood stream – and you know what happens to a house repaired with straw.

It is for this reason that one successful slimming diet, the Lindlahr, should not be maintained for more than two weeks. In this period most people can lose 14 pounds. It is based on Dr Lindlahr's theory that some foods are 'catabolic' that is to say the body uses more calories in digesting them than the food itself provides in energy calories. A head of lettuce, say, may supply 20 calories and cost the body 30 for its disposal. This theory is not accepted by many medical men who point out that Dr Lindlahr's slimming diet, while high in bulk, is very low in calories, providing no more than about 600 a day.

He suggests a glass of fruit juice and one whole fruit with as much of the skin and pith as possible for breakfast. For lunch a large salad, raw, with lemon dressing, two cooked vegetables and a serving of fruit, preferably uncooked, certainly without sugar. The same for dinner.

At one meal add cottage cheese or a small portion of fatless fish or meat.

This is a good healthy clean-out diet but, as we said, it is too low on protein and also on fats to maintain for more than two weeks. But if you have more than 14 lb. to lose it can be alternated with a low carbohydrate gram diet which produces, perhaps, a slower weight loss but provides proteins and fats that the body needs. However this, too, is short of some essentials like the vitamins and minerals from fruits, and too high in saturated fats for those with a high serum cholesterol.

Instead of counting calories you count carbohydrate grams and for this you will probably have to buy, or find in a book, a gram counter. It has been agreed that most people can lose weight on a diet which allows for no more than 60 grams of carbohydrate a day.

There are very few carbohydrate grams in meat, fish, eggs, cheese, butter, cream, vegetable oil and, on a low carbohydrate gram diet, these can be taken freely. Green leafy vegetables, citrus fruits, strawberries, rhubarb are fairly low but most other fruits and vegetables must be taken cautiously. Anything containing flour or sugar is practically ruled out by the fact that it gives too many grams for the amount of food value you get from it. However some dry wine or spirits, tea or coffee with cream and a sweetener (no milk or sugar) are allowed. Sugar substitutes (with the exception of sorbitol), and a small amount of starch reduced bread or biscuits may be used.

Once you have lost what you set out to lose the problem is to maintain the weight loss. It is no good losing 50 lb. in a year – and gaining 110.

Most people tend to gain weight after the age of 25 or 30, not necessarily because they eat more and exercise less, though this can happen, but because their needs decrease by about 1 per cent per year. This works out at $2\frac{1}{2}$ lb. a year or 25 lb. in 10 years – as Dr Herbert Pollack, Metabolic specialist, recently pointed out. His solution was to decrease one's food intake gradually, or to add some simple daily exercise.

Easier said than done. It's not easy to add 30 minutes extra walking daily: 10 or 15 minutes home exercises a day will do it if you haven't been doing them before. Or you can cut out something you have regularly been eating: a sweet biscuit, a cup of cocoa at bedtime, sweets at any time.

It's *not* easy. Some can do it one way and some another and some say they can't do it at all – but they'd better. Added weight as you get older puts an added burden on the heart – and on the eye of the beholder should you happen to be vain – and who isn't?

To re-educate your eating habits, then, you can substitute:

1. A non-calorie sweetener for sugar.
2. Clear soup for thickened soups, gravies or sauces with poultry, meat and fish.
3. Fruit for chocolates or sweets.
4. Protein crispbread or nothing served with your meals.
5. Cabbage, broccoli, string beans, sprouts or any leafy vegetables for root or pod vegetables.
6. Vegetable sticks, hard-boiled eggs, fish or cheese without crackers for pastry type canapes.
7. Dry drinks for sweet ones.

As well, buy a weighing machine, note your weight daily in a notebook and take your vital statistics – bust, waist, tummy and hips – once a week. Over the weeks and months and even years this will be a useful guide and prevent you from straying too far from the straight and narrow figure.

However, don't cut out all your favourite foods at one fell swoop, or you may end up with a terrific gorge. Re-train your appetite so that in the end, even if you fall for the gorge, it will be disappointing. To start, take half size portions of your particular weakness. Let's say this is ice-cream. If you are on the low gram diet you're allowed cream so make the ice-cream yourself using thick cream, a sweetener instead of sugar, a permitted fruit – strawberries, for instance.

Start your main meal with a salad. These not only take the edge off your appetite but provide, along with their bulk, many essential vitamins and minerals. There are lots of ways of varying salads and making them interesting. Buy a vegetable grater and you can put in grated cheese, nuts, carrots, cabbage; a slicer (which often comes with the same little gadget: one of these is a Mouligrater No. 2 but there are others) can cut cucumber and onion slices very fine. Another little gadget (a Parsmint) will chop up mint, parsley or most other herbs that you can grow in your garden or on your window ledge. For a dressing use an unsaturated vegetable oil: safflower, sunflower, soya, corn or peanut. Combine it with cider vinegar, a small amount of honey and any dried or fresh herbs. Unsaturated vegetable oil has many virtues, one of which is that it helps the body throw off excess water which often causes a swelling of the tissues and adds to the appearance of obesity.

Eat lots of fish. It is not only much lower in calories than meat, its fat is of the unsaturated kind. Also it contains iodine, good for the gland which regulates the rate you burn your food. With insufficient iodine this gland becomes sluggish and your metabolism slows down.

Ever since overweight became a problem of overcivilisation, all the nutrition and diet experts in the world have been devising newer and better methods of slimming. Many of them offer good props for flagging determination and many suggest goals which make it easier. But, sad to say, by whatever route they reach their destination, the conclusion is that one must

    1. Take in less food than is used up in energy.

    2. Cut down, or cut out, high, processed carbohydrates.

INSTRUCTION 21

IMPORTANT POINTS TO REMEMBER IN POSTURAL TRAINING AND HOME TREATMENT

1. **Active Alerted Balanced Posture** must be practised whenever you are standing:
    (a) Is your weight on the outer side of your feet with the toes gripping the floor?
    (b) Are your knees slightly bent?
    (c) Is your abdomen being held up at all times?
    (d) Are your buttocks tucked under and in slight contraction?
    (e) Are you standing as tall as possible, with the chin tucked in and the shoulders held up and slightly forward?
2. At rest, either sitting or lying, you should be in the Passive Supported Position (Figs. **21**, 1 and **21**, 2).
3. When you lift, pull or push anything, remember two important points:
    (a) The load, the force and the lever must be as nearly as possible in line with one another (Fig. **21**, 3).
    (b) The 'activator' muscles must be assisted by the 'synergist' muscles, acting on the 'prime fixers', and the prime fixing level must be locked (Fig. **21**, 4).
4. Home Treatment must be carried out Religiously, Regularly, Resolutely (even if somewhat reluctantly!) at least twice each day while a pathological condition is present, and once a day after it has disappeared.
5. If pain and stiffness persist for more than a few days, or if a limp develops, take it seriously and consult your doctor at once.

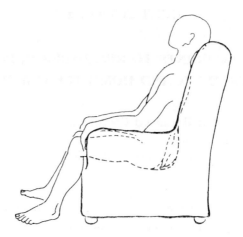

FIG. **21**, 1
Passive Supported Posture Sitting.

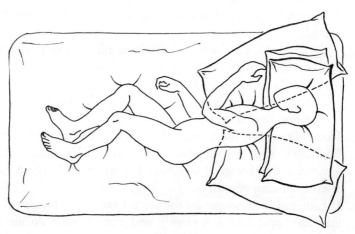

FIG. **21**, 2
Passive Supported Posture, lying with the joints in a neutral position.

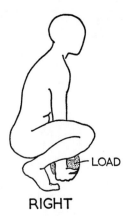

RIGHT

FIG. 21, 3
The right way to lift weights.

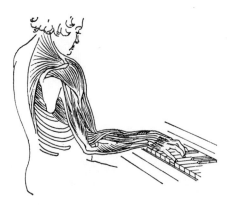

FIG. 21, 4
Pianist in the act of playing showing the activating groups of muscles controlling
the fingers, the synergistic groups controlling the wrist, elbow and shoulder
joints, and the prime fixer groups controlling the shoulder girdle.

INDEX

PRINTED BY GEORGE OUTRAM & CO. LTD., 36 TAY STREET, PERTH, SCOTLAND